INTIMATE ATTACHMENTS

⤳ INTIMATE ATTACHMENTS

Toward a New Self Psychology

MORTON SHANE
ESTELLE SHANE
MARY GALES

THE GUILFORD PRESS
New York   London

© 1997 The Guilford Press
A Division of Guilford Publications, Inc.
72 Spring Street, New York, NY 10012
www.guilford.com

Printed in the United States of America

This book is printed on acid-free paper.

Last digit is print number: 9 8 7 6 5 4 3 2 1

Library of Congress Cataloging-in-Publication Data

Shane, Morton.
    Intimate attachments: toward a new self psychology / Morton
Shane, Estelle Shane, Mary Gales.
      p.   cm.
    Includes bibliographical references and index.
    ISBN 1-57230-270-4
    1. Self psychology. 2. Psychotherapist and patient.
3. Intimacy (Psychology) 4. Attachment behavior.
I. Shane, Estelle. II. Gales, Mary. III. Title.
RC489.S43S52   1997
616.89'14—dc21   97-37393
                                                      CIP

∿ *To our three children, Russ Shane,
David Shane, and Ben Gales*

Acknowledgments

We want to acknowledge first of all the Institute of Contemporary Psychoanalysis. In the atmosphere of academic freedom and innovative psychoanalytic thinking that this institute embodies, we were able to teach, supervise, and pursue our ideas without restraint. We are grateful as well to the faculty and candidates of this institute for their willingness to provide a forum for sharing and shaping our views in many contexts.

We want to acknowledge individually a few of the many people who were helpful to us in this venture. Keith Valone worked with us collaboratively in an early effort to integrate developmental systems and attachment theory. Lou Breger read an initial draft of this work, offering many helpful suggestions. Barbara Breger, with her capacity to understand what we are about, provided us with the quote from George Eliot that appears in Chapter 3. Without the help of Jane Mason we could not have met the necessary deadlines with a feeling of competence and completeness. Most centrally, we want to acknowledge the invaluable, dedicated, and patient work of our editor at The Guilford Press, Kitty Moore, who put up with a good deal in order to help us make this book more readable and accessible.

Finally, we want to express our gratitude to our families for their encouragement, support, and forbearance: Harold and Mildred Heser, Ben Gales, Delaine and Russ Shane, Constance and David Shane, Jennifer Shane, and Jeffrey Shane.

Contents

INTIMATE ATTACHMENTS

Introduction

Human beings who are loved and responded to by caring others acquire a consolidated self over the course of their development and a capacity for pleasurable intimacy with others. Trauma, in the form of parental failure or constitutional difficulties in the child, disrupts this progressive and interdependent process toward self- and self-with-other consolidation. As a result, the vital experience of the self coming into being and being in connection is impeded. From our perspective, psychoanalysis carries with it the potential to provide a positive new experience for the individual who suffered trauma to the self in this way. Our book is an effort to describe this process through theoretical and clinical means.

We will both explain and illustrate our approach, comparing and contrasting it to the multiplicity of models that already exist in the pluralistic community in which we live and practice. We want to clarify the particular aspects of our framework, show their origins in the psychoanalytic writings of others and in relevant findings from other fields, and articulate our own innovations. Our approach unremittingly emphasizes the importance and value of positive new experience in the clinical situation. We have derived this focus from our combined knowledge of self psychology, attachment literature, infant research, trauma studies, developmental systems research, and brain research. We apply a nonlinear dynamic systems model to create a unity of these various strands.

ELEMENTS OF OUR MODEL

In this chapter we outline the essential features of our framework, but first we offer a brief clinical vignette that highlights one of these features, the positive new experience in the psychoanalytic situation.

An analyst sought consultation with a supervisor because he was puzzled. He complained that he was unable to find signs of transference with his patient. He felt like a failure as an analyst, but yet as a therapist he felt like a success. His patient was doing famously, feeling both grateful and loving toward her analyst. Yet the analyst feared that something must be wrong. He must have been missing something important, for how could this be analysis?

The treatment had begun with the patient describing a troubled relationship with her mother, and her description gradually unfolded into a horrendous account of her childhood. It featured a mother so out of control that once in a state of rage, she attempted to smother the patient in her bed with a pillow. The patient's life was saved only through the intervention of her maternal grandmother who came upon the scene unexpectedly and pulled the mother off of the child. The mother was sent away by the grandmother for several weeks until the mother could regain some measure of composure. However, repeated episodes of dangerously aggressive attacks continued throughout the patient's childhood. A marker of the most extreme incident— the attempted smothering—was the patient's mysterious, lifelong inability to sleep with a pillow in her bed. This connection was made through a sudden insight on the patient's part, bringing with it conviction of the emotional veracity of her heretofore disavowed memory.

Such revelations continued throughout the first 18 months of the patient's analysis, with the analyst doing no more than listening, making appropriate connections, resonating with the patient's affects, and consolidating the patient's sense of self and evolving life narrative. Throughout this period the analyst puzzled over what, if any, analytic function he was providing, with the puzzle abating somewhat when the patient said, quite spontaneously during one session, "This experience with you is the first time in my life I ever have felt safe." With this moving declaration, the analyst at least had some idea that something important was going on, but he was nevertheless left with the nagging question, But is this *analysis*? And if it is analysis, how can it be, with so little transference experience and so much positive new experience that for the patient was different than she had ever before encountered? It did not seem as if the patient experienced her analyst in old conflictual ways stemming from the past, which analysis is customarily supposed to address. So what was he missing?

The supervisor helped this analyst to understand that by viewing the patient from a perspective different from the more conventional one the analyst had been using, this patient, suffering from trauma that had seriously compromised self-development, could now be seen as benefiting from a positive new experience in the analysis. That is, the patient was relating to her analyst as a novel other in her life, in a new, protective, intimately attached, and vitalizing relationship, which in fact had been in place virtually throughout the analysis. The traumatic past, although not lived out in a transference relationship with the analyst, that is, although not being experienced with him directly, was nevertheless very much part of the analytic work, both in the form it took in the patient's memories, and in the contrast it offered to the patient's present feelings of safety, and security with the analyst as a positive new other.

We are proposing in this book a framework in which self, trauma, and positive new experience are conceptualized as focal elements. The positive new experience in analysis encompasses that process of self fully coming into being as a consolidated self, and comfortably and safely coming into connection with the analyst as an intimate other. Nonlinear dynamic systems theory serves as a guiding organization for our framework. We have found that a systems approach accurately captures the complexities of human development and explains its multifaceted manifestations in the clinical situation. In our experience, this guiding organization can offer therapists the maximum of freedom, creativity, and spontaneity to help their patients recover from the varieties of trauma from which they suffer and for which they seek help.

We identify then, certain desirable, optimal outcomes both in development and in the clinical situation. We assume that given an appropriately responsive environment and adequate constitutional endowment, self- and self-with-other consolidation will emerge. It is precisely these optimal conditions and these optimal outcomes that we try to conceptualize and delineate in our framework.

We conceptualize development as a progression toward such consolidation of self and self with other. We conceptualize trauma as those circumstances that cause an interference with self- and self-with-other consolidation so that development is disrupted. This understanding of trauma includes the outcomes of both environmental deficiency, which may take the form of neglect, loss, and active abuse, and constitutional deficiency. In response to these traumatic circumstances, self-protective coping mechanisms are adopted by the individual, which represent the best and most adaptive response available at the time. This adaptive response allows the person the greatest degree of self-preservation and attachment to the needed other. We think of these responses as self-protective strategies rather than as pathological defenses because we would contend that at the time such strategies were developed by the child, they represented survival not pathology. Nevertheless, however adaptive these strategies may have been, they did interfere with development toward self-consolidation and the capacity to turn to significant others for needed safety, security, and self-regulation. Psychoanalysis thus becomes a way to reactivate that developmental course toward self- and self-with-other consolidation that trauma had disrupted. This reactivation constitutes positive new experience, a concept central to therapeutic action in our framework.

Dimensions of Intimacy

We begin with the elaboration of two elements vital to the achievement of positive new experience. The first element is the *dimensions of intimacy* that emerge in the psychoanalytic situation, that is, how patient and analyst connect in the dyad and how each lives with and experiences the other within their connection. We believe that the self evolves and consolidates in development through these forms of connectedness. A secure base is formed in the analytic relationship, out of which, in a spiral fashion, the patient's self can consolidate. We posit two dimensions of intimacy which together capture the human relatedness inherent in psychoanalytic progress in our model. The first is the *self with self-transforming other* dimension, concerned with how the dyad is used to regulate and transform the patient toward coming more fully into being as a person in his or her own right. The second is the *self with interpersonal-sharing other* dimension, concerned with how the dyad is used to create a capacity to be with an other in mutual sharing and mutual appreciation, that is, being more fully in connection. The analyst's conception of the dimension active in the dyad informs his or her listening position, which we view as a metaphor for the diverse ways that patient and analyst relate and communicate with one another. The dimension of intimacy present thus helps to guide the analyst in listening and responding, in being with the patient, and it provides some orientation for when and what the analyst shares. The dimension of intimacy helps determine when and how the analyst answers questions, and whether or not the analyst participates in certain experiences with the patient, such as whether to receive or even give gifts, whether to provide extra-analytic contact, or give advice, or decide to hold a patient's hand.

The dimensions of intimacy are described in terms of how the patient experiences the analyst, so that the "self" in these designations is the patient's self, with the analyst designated as either the other that serves to transform the self, or as the other that serves to share intimacy interpersonally with the self. In the self with self-transforming other dimension of intimacy, the analyst is experienced by the patient as an other who provides significant functions for the self, including self-regulation, self-affirmation, self-delineation, and self-state stabilization. This category of relatedness owes its conceptual origins both to Kohut's (1977) selfobject and Stern's (1985) self-regulating other, with specific attributes emphasized from our developmental systems self psychology perspective, which clearly distinguishes ours from these earlier concepts. The attributes that differentiate the self-transforming other from the selfobject are as follows:

1. The nature of this relatedness is essentially positive, so that even when, as is common, the patient is experiencing negative or dysphoric affect, the analyst attempts to provide a consistent ambiance of hope, optimism, and safety that the patient may or may not be able to appreciate or to reflect upon at that moment in time. The analyst who follows our guidelines does not aim to frustrate, however optimally, as does the analyst who follows Kohut's guidelines.

2. We emphasize, as distinct from the unidirectionality inherent in the selfobject concept, the ever-present mutual influence and bidirectionality of interaction in the dyad. Moreover, we believe it is this very mutuality and bidirectionality inevitably present in the dyad that provides one avenue for the positive new experience we contend is essential to psychoanalytic cure. We argue that the analyst always goes beyond empathy and beyond the understanding emergent from that empathy, through the action of conveying, even without meaning to, an equally significant communication of his or her own, deriving from the unavoidable, nonverbal, affectful feeling state evoked in the analyst by the patient in the moment. That is, when a patient feels dysphoric affects such as hopelessness and despair, or anger and disappointment, the analyst does inevitably feel something in response, and does inevitably communicate in some way and to some significant degree whatever those feelings are. It is best in our view if the response that is thus conveyed is one that not only communicates the empathic resonance with the patient's emotional state that is so important for connection, but presents an additional perspective belonging to the analyst of an inner, unspoken attempt to sustain an

optimistic balance. This is an instance of positive new experience in the analytic situation, one that moves beyond empathy and understanding.

3. An attribute distinguishing the self-transforming other from the selfobject is that we conceptualize as *always* present in the self-transforming other concept the patient's sustained awareness of the other as an important presence, though the use to which that other is put excludes the importance of the other's subjectivity, motives, intentions, and/or emotions, except insofar as they are experienced by the patient as operating in the service of the patient's own well-being.

4. The experience of the self-transforming other is postulated to be a positive new experience, not based on templates from the past, thus it is neither a transference nor a transference-like manifestation.

5. The self-transforming other differs from Stern's (1985) self-regulating other because it offers the patient many other transformative experiences for the self, rather than just regulation. Moreover, it goes beyond the preverbal self-with-other intimacy of the core self described by Stern to include aspects of Stern's intersubjective and verbal self-with-other intimacy.

In contrast, in the self with interpersonal-sharing other dimension of intimacy, the analyst is experienced by the patient as an other whose self, motives, intentions, emotions, and subjectivity are appreciated for their own sake, and not just in relation to the patient's needs, as pertains in the self-transforming dimension. The patient's sense of intimacy is based on interpersonal sharing, which includes subjective, intersubjective, and procedural sharing and other nonsubjective experiences of self with other. This dimension of intimacy encompasses experiences of shared humanity, heightened mutuality, affection, liking, and even love between analyst and patient. Each person in the dyad is vitally interested in the other. This shared intimate experience is not always equal. Most importantly, the patient's development is always maintained as central to the interaction between them.

Relational Configurations

The second element vital to the achievement of positive new experience is the concept we refer to as the *relational configuration*. We conceptualize three relational configurations: *old self with old other, old self with new other,* and *new self with new other.* These describe the influence of the traumatic past on the organization of present-day lived experience, and the struggle to overcome in analysis the pernicious influence of old, constricting patterns that keep the patient locked in that traumatic past. The relational configurations we describe encompass the meliorative trajectory of development leading out of repetitive patterns, which rob the patient of benefiting from and enjoying the present, toward a new life less dominated by the painful past. The past is not totally lost, of course, but the patient gains an ability to distinguish that past from the present in a way that is flexible, adaptive, and creative, enhancing the patient's sense of reality, and of being real. This trajectory of developmental progression defines an aspect of the forward movement in both development in general and analysis in particular. This movement is toward consolidation of the self and consolidation of the intimate tie to the other, toward the self coming into being and being in connection. As such, the configurations move along a continuum from old to new, from childhood to adulthood, from suffering to health, or, to paraphrase Robert Stoller (1975), from trauma to triumph.

The first relational configuration is the old self with old other patient–analyst relational configuration. In this configuration, the patient experiences both self and analyst in a repetition of patterns categorized predominantly on the basis of traumatic, past lived experience, patterns that encompass the old, traumatized self along with the old, traumatogenic other. In this configuration, the present either does not exist or has only minimal impact on shaping the patient's experience of the analyst. *This configuration represents transference in our model.*

In the second relational configuration, the old self with new other patient–analyst relational configuration, the patient continues to categorize himself or herself predominantly in old, traumatized ways but is beginning to experience the analyst as different from past traumatogenic figures.

The third configuration is the new self with new other patient–analyst relational configuration. In this configuration, the patient categorizes both himself or herself and the analyst predominantly in novel ways not based on the traumatogenic past. In this last relational configuration, current, novel, in-the-moment perception and experience predominates. The relational configuration that is presently operating helps to guide the analyst's listening and responding, and provides some orientation for recognizing and working with the patient's currently maladaptive, outdated self-protective strategies, for recognizing the contribution of the past to present-day organization of lived experience, and for facilitating the developmental progression from past to present toward consolidation of the self and consolidation of the tie to the other. Such consolidation is marked by a new sense of past, present, and future as continuous, and a new capacity to locate oneself in time with full access to one's emotional experiences, all embedded in a rich, comprehensive, coherent life narrative. The optimal outcome is also evidenced in the patient's clear sense of direction, reality, motivation, and originality in designing his or her life, and in choosing partners who are loving and avoiding those who are not.

If we take the case with which we opened this chapter, we can conceptualize the patient's experience in a new way. Far from being "not in analysis," this patient was deeply involved in a relationship with the analyst, which functioned in a new self with new other configuration. This is different from most analytic understanding. This supervisor had conceptual room for a new, never-before experienced sense of safety, that is, a positive new experience of self with other, one never before lived through, one not based on old relational patterns, one not considered to be a gratification of longings either fulfilled or unfulfilled from the patient's past, one not conceptualized as transference. Moreover, this supervisor did not feel that everything meliorative in treatment had to be experienced in the transference. He also did not believe that all relationships with the analyst have to be punctuated either by negative experiences or by disruptions and repairs if there is to be a significant developmental advance toward cure. In this supervisor's view, then, this positive new experience constituted analysis.

This vignette also illustrates an instance of "nonlinearity" in our framework, with the analysis beginning and proceeding in a new–new relational configuration, one that could not have been predicted to emerge at the onset of treatment, and one that continues unbroken to the present. Any patient–analyst relational configuration, or any sequence of such configurations, may arise in the analytic system at any given time. That is, an old self with old other configuration may arise as the predominant relational pattern first in the analysis, or an old self with new other configuration, or, as in the illustration given, a new self with new other configuration may emerge first. It is the system itself, then, and not any particular configuration, or any particular order of configuration, that we identify as psychoanalytic.

Several points must be highlighted. First, it is not necessary that other configurations arise in the system between analyst and patient for it to be considered a viable developmental systems self psychology approach. Second, although the analysis seems to have begun in and continues to progress in a new–new relational configuration, this may not be the only configuration that will arise in the treatment. At any time, another configuration may emerge, ascending to the prominence of a relatively stable pattern (a *deep attractor state* in nonlinear dynamic systems terms) that we refer to with the term "relational configuration." Most importantly, if an analysis remains persistently in a new–new relational configuration, it does not mean that it is not an analysis, nor that important material has been overlooked or omitted in the patient–analyst relationship.

OVERVIEW OF THE BOOK

In the chapters that follow, we will elaborate on our developmental systems self psychology framework and its clinical applications. Specifically, the next chapter considers the essential features and origins of the model. Chapter 3 addresses the two dimensions of intimacy. Chapter 4 reexamines and redefines transference. Chapter 5 describes the three relational configurations. Chapter 6 is composed of more extended clinical applications of the concepts of dimensions of intimacy and relational configurations. Finally, Chapters 7 through 9 address the application of our model across the lifespan from infancy through adulthood.

CHAPTER TWO

Essential Features
and Origins of the Model

In this chapter we begin by describing the origins of our model. We review first the two main psychoanalytic theories on which our work is based, self psychology and attachment studies. We then discuss those aspects we draw on from developmental systems research and brain research. The postulates we derive from all of these sources, along with the innovations we devise based on our own clinical work, are then integrated through the application of nonlinear dynamic systems understanding. This integration serves to create a developmental systems self psychology based on the self coming into being and being in connection.

CRUCIAL ELEMENTS FROM SELF PSYCHOLOGY: KOHUT AND HIS FOLLOWERS

In identifying our conceptual roots, we begin with our connection to self psychology. Self psychology encompasses several very different perspectives (M. Shane & Shane, 1993), reflective of the general pluralism present today in psychoanalysis. What most obviously continues to distinguish self psychology from the majority of psychoanalytic thought is its consistent focus on the centrality of the self.

The currently recognized, divergent self psychological perspectives include essentially three models: (1) the *self–selfobject matrix model*, whose proponents (e.g., Goldberg, 1978; Ornstein & Ornstein, 1980, M. Tolpin 1986; P. Tolpin, 1985; Wolf, 1988) largely follow Kohut's (1971, 1977) original vision; (2) *intersubjectivity theory*, whose proponents (e.g., Stolorow, Brandchaft, & Atwood, 1987) focus on the

organizing principles that emerge in the confluence of shared subjectivities; and (3) *motivational systems and affect theory*, whose proponents
(e.g., Lichtenberg, Lachmann, & Fosshage, 1992) emphasize the function served in the dyad by the emergent motivational system and its
identifying affect state. These three perspectives, as well as the developmental systems self psychology perspective to be presented in this
book, are all organized around Kohut's emphasis on self as central.

It seems important to remind ourselves of the context in which
Kohut (1971, 1977, 1984) wrote, a context that persists today. Kohut
generated his own theories within a scientific milieu wherein ideas of
normal development based on prospective and normative infant observation, as put forward by John Bowlby (1969, 1973, 1988, 1989),
Mary Ainsworth (1982, 1985), and James and Joyce Robertson (1969),
were being pitted against retrospective and pathomorphic views found
in the Freudian and Kleinian perspectives. Hence, Kohut wrote at a
time when studies on attachment, the nature of relatedness, the
traumatic etiology of much mental suffering, and new ways of understanding how treatment helps were very much in process. He simultaneously influenced and was influenced by these contemporaneous
currents, creating a unique theory that itself has enjoyed both wide
influence and serious challenges from his followers. This led to the
current multifaceted self psychological scene, in which there yet
remains an adherence, more or less, to specific aspects of Kohut's
legacy.

Kohut's theoretical and clinical contributions may be addressed
in terms of particular basic assumptions drawn from the body of his
work, which have informed the various self psychologies. These have
been extended and expanded by different theorists. In this section we
will explore each of these assumptions.

The first assumption is the application of the empathic-introspec-
tive mode as largely defining and delimiting the domain of psychoanalytic inquiry. Kohut (1971, 1977, 1984) identified empathy as the
principal source of psychoanalytic data gathering, as a powerful bond
in development from infancy on, and as a means of therapeutic action
in the analytic situation. Some of the current trends in self psychology,
including our own model, amend this view both by adding to it. For
example, Fosshage (in press) identified an additional listening perspective, which he termed "other-centered listening," that is, listening that
is based in the analyst's own perspective. This listening perspective
serves as an addition to Kohut's concept of listening to the patient
from the patient's perspective. As another example, Strenger (1991)

puts forward the concept of external coherence which focuses on the use of disciplines ancillary to psychoanalysis as both source and check on the value of data obtained in the psychoanalytic situation. As an illustration of the use of external coherence, we can cite Lichtenberg (1989) who supports his motivational systems conceptualization with ample data drawn from relevant infant research and neurophysiological studies.

A second basic assumption of Kohut's (1971, 1977, 1984) work includes both the lifelong need of the individual for selfobject functions and the varieties of selfobject transferences performing these functions, as may be seen in the psychoanalytic situation. Selfobject functions serve to develop, sustain, and regulate the self, and include the provision of soothing, calming, and admiring, as well as of a source for idealizing and of being just like an other. These functions were categorized by Kohut in terms of three selfobject transferences: mirroring, idealizing, and alter ego. The selfobject bond that forms between patient and analyst in the psychoanalytic situation can be understood as the form that attachment motivation takes in Kohut's theory, a form that focuses on important functions and experiences provided for the self by the selfobject, but that does not encompass the full bidirectionality implied in Bowlby's attachment theory (e.g., 1988, 1989), in infant research (e.g., Stern, 1985; Beebe & Lachmann, 1992), and in some other models of self psychology, including our own. In addition, in the developmental systems self psychology perspective we present, we focus on an aspect that remains largely unarticulated within Kohut's concept of the self–selfobject relationship, but that we see as a salient contributor to psychoanalytic process: namely, the ongoing, sustaining, facilitating relationship, which we reconceptualize as the positive new experience contained within the patient–analyst connection, and which itself, in our model, is a major contributor to therapeutic action and to desired outcome.

A third assumption is that the psychoanalytic process carries, along with insight, a significant developmental power and thrust. Thus for Kohut (1971, 1977, 1984), and for most self psychologists, psychoanalysis itself is a developmental experience in which the infant–caregiver, self–selfobject matrix serves as the analogue of mental health for the patient–analyst, self–selfobject matrix.

The fourth assumption centers on the importance of optimal frustration, that is, frustration of the patient's need that is not so intense that fragmentation of the self occurs as a consequence. Kohut believed that through optimal frustration psychological structure ensues, a notion that has been challenged in terms of its developmental accuracy, power, and singularity. Infant research and attachment theory have shown other interactions in addition to frustration that support self-development. These interactions include affect integration (Socarides & Stolorow, 1984–1985); optimal responsiveness (Bacal, 1985; Terman, 1988), ongoing regulation (Stern, 1985; Beebe & Lachmann, 1992); heightened affective moments (Stern, 1985; Pine, 1990; Beebe & Lachmann, 1992); and interpersonal-sharing intimacy (E. Shane, Gales, & Shane, 1995). Thus for many self psychologists, the concept of optimal frustration is not adequate to explain learning and developmental progression either in life or in the clinical situation.

The fifth assumption we draw from Kohut's (1971, 1977, 1984) work is that of viewing destructive aggression not as primary drive, but as a response secondary to frustration. This destructive aggression is often understood as narcissistic rage. Similarly, in our model, destructive aggression is essentially reactive, with the intensity either heightened or diminished by individual constitutional endowment. We add that destructive aggression, where prominent in the person, is most often understood to have been evoked in traumatogenic lived experience.

The sixth assumption concerns the concept of defense as primarily self-preservative. We view trauma, including passive neglect as well as active abuse, as being connected to the elaboration of so-called defenses. These represent the best possible self-protective strategies for the individual at that time in development, serving the child's adaptational needs in an inadequate, unresponsive, or abusive milieu. These self-protective strategies are then preserved as patterns of expectation or relatedness that come to organize the self, and that involve patterns of self with important other in interaction.

Finally, as a seventh assumption we consider that Kohut's (1984) separation of the interpretative act into its component parts of understanding and explaining opens up interpretation to the developmental possibilities inherent for the patient in the experience of being both understood and enlightened. In Kohut's definition, the understanding phase of interpretation refers to the process in which the analyst empathetically articulates the patient's subjective experience. The explaining phase refers to the analyst's addition of dynamic and genetic connections to this empathic understanding. As we have stated, we conceptualize therapeutic action as going beyond understanding and explaining to include additional forms of positive new experience.

In addition to Kohut's theoretical contributions, Kohut's personal creativity and the way in which he conducted his life remain an inspiration in our own approach. Kohut exercised both courage and originality in following his clinical impressions. His letters (Cocks, 1994) provide many instances of his ability to go his own way and to allow others to do the same. For example, as an influential member of the American Psychoanalytic Association, he was consistently on the side of academic freedom and against the tight hierarchical control exercised by most psychoanalytic institutes in this country vis-à-vis the appointment of training and supervising analysts. He took a forthright position on the side of lay analysis at a time when such training was highly unpopular. He supported as well the equal status of child analysis in the International Psychoanalytic Association, a stance that was also considered less than acceptable by his contemporaries. These positions, which demonstrate Kohut's courage and capacity for independent thought, are important for the valuable insight they provide into the man Kohut was and the man he was to become, but we include this discussion and the example that follows for another reason. The example provides a perspective on Kohut's overall attitude not only philosophically but clinically, focusing as it does on the capacity for empathic involvement with the other even under the most trying of circumstances. This capacity is of central significance to Kohut's theory, as well as to the influence Kohut had on the development of our framework.

In 1965, when Kohut was past-president of the American Psychoanalytic Association, a particularly difficult situation came to his attention. Victor Rosen, the current president of the Association, had disgraced himself in the eyes of his colleagues by planning to marry a candidate-analysand. Kohut wrote to Victor Rosen:

> As an individual I would grant you that it is courageous to go counter to established attitudes if one is convinced that one is right; and I have no doubt that you are convinced of it. But your personal conviction and your personal courage are not the issue at stake while you are the president [of the American Psychoanalytic Association]. To many . . . your actions will imply a loosening of the basic ethical obligation of analysts: not to make use of their patient's emotional attachment for any purpose other than to enlarge their mastery over themselves through insight. . . . Despite my overriding concern for psychoanalysis, I wish you well as a person. . . . I truly hope for your happiness and your inner balance. (in Cocks, 1994, p. 129)

This letter is quoted here, as we said, to illustrate Kohut's exercise of empathy in the face of a situation that challenges his clear ethical position that one should not exploit one's patient, and the dialectical tension created in Kohut by the other side in this situation, namely, Kohut's respect for the subjective perspective of the other. Kohut also maintained the theoretical and clinical stance that one cannot simply judge an other from outside the empathic position, even in a matter as grave in its implications as this one. It is important to note that Kohut was at that time on the threshold of officially launching self psychology, already having written drafts of "Forms and Transformations of Narcissism" (1968), and on the way to writing his revolutionary book, *The Analysis of the Self* (1971). Kohut was also at the pinnacle of his political prominence in organized psychoanalysis as past president of the American Psychoanalytic Association and was contemplating running for president of the International Psychoanalytic Association. He could well have taken scornful umbrage at Victor Rosen's transgression of accepted, well-thought-out analytic standards, avoiding possible criticism by seeming to be in any way equivocal on this point. Yet, even under such pressing circumstances, he had room for contemplating and appreciating an other's inner state, and could leave open the possibility that although from the point of view of Kohut's own ideals and values, Rosen was wrong, from Victor Rosen's point of view, Rosen must have felt right for himself in some profound and personal way.

Our point here is that not only did Kohut teach that the analyst should respect the patient's assertions as accurate reflections of the patient's sense of reality, even when the analyst's sense of reality differed markedly, but that Kohut was capable of living his extraclinical life in the same manner. The incident illustrates also our contention that the man and his theory are closely connected, that the theory and the man who espouses the theory match, and that, finally, the person of the analyst has great importance in the clinical work he does.

A further implication for Kohut's psychoanalytic stance should be mentioned: While he could, and should, understand, respect, and appreciate an other's point of view, he would not abandon his own view, nor withhold his own personal opinion. This balance in self psychology is too often lost, or at the least misunderstood, by those who see self psychology as teaching an unvarying adherence to the patient's subjective perspective. One of the contributions we want to honor in this volume, and hope thereby to retain from Kohut's legacy, is just this balance between open-mindedness toward others and assertion of oneself, the courage to speak one's own mind at the same time that one respectfully listens to an other's, always holding open the possibility that you could be wrong and that those who hold alternative views could be right in some profound way.

ATTACHMENT THEORY: JOHN BOWLBY'S WORK

At this point we will introduce basic theoretical and clinical assumptions distilled from John Bowlby's (1969, 1973, 1988, 1989) significant and unique contributions to psychoanalytic understanding, contributions that are particularly pertinent to our own approach. We will begin with a brief look into Bowlby's professional life because his experience influenced his theory from the start, keeping him from ever fully ascribing to traditional psychoanalytic conceptualizations. Like Kohut, Bowlby was consistently able to follow his own clinical impressions, challenging accepted theory and ultimately devising his own. He began with first-hand, clinically based, nonpsychoanalytic experience with children, experience that would not permit him, once initiated into psychoanalytic training, to accept received analytic wisdom, but instead would require him to confront and modify what had gone before in psychoanalytic thought.

The entire period he was in medical school and analytic training, Bowlby worked with emotionally disturbed children and their families. This direct clinical involvement facilitated his understanding of the importance of real life experience and trauma in the etiology of psychological illness, particularly the deleterious effects of maternal deprivation on the emotional health of infants and children. Yet, at the same time, his training at the British Psychoanalytic Institute was teaching him the opposite. Based on the theories of Sigmund Freud and Melanie Klein, he was told that the infant's and child's inborn drives and fantasy life were more directly influential in the inner world of the individual than was the individual's lifetime of interpersonal encounters with significant others. Added to these psychological streams of thought was Anna Freud's (1966) concept of "cupboard love," that is, that the child becomes attached to whomever feeds him or her. Moreover, this particular connection, the deep attachment of the child to the caregiver, was conceptualized as a phase-specific requirement, that is, a requirement specific and appropriate to early childhood, but outgrown as the child undergoes libidinal development in the direction of independence and autonomy. Such teachings were in direct conflict with his clinical experience, and this conflict brought Bowlby into a significant struggle with the psychoanalytic world of his day.

His supervision with Melanie Klein is an example of Bowlby's professional experience coming in conflict with his education, as he revealed in a lecture on the origins of attachment theory (1990). As a young analyst in training, he presented to Mrs. Klein a child patient whose mother was psychotic. Klein told Bowlby that the mother's psychological problems were irrelevant to his patient's difficulties, that the little boy's pathology derived from his internal unconscious conflicts and fantasies. This dissonant comment from Melanie Klein greatly contrasted not only with Bowlby's first-hand, nonanalytic work with children, but also with his growing awareness of experimental work in other areas, including studies conducted in the 1940s and 1950s on children's reactions to loss and subsequent mourning (Spitz, 1946; Spitz & Cobliner, 1965; Robertson & Robertson, 1969; Robertson & Bowlby, 1952); ethological studies on imprinting in animals (Lorenz, 1957); and the effects on primates of maternal deprivation (Harlow & Harlow, 1965).

All of this knowledge convinced Bowlby (1988) that actual happenings matter much in the psychological life of the individual. Bowlby postulated that attachment is a fundamental motivation in its own right, leading him to speculate that separation anxiety and mourning are responses to the loss of the attachment figure, and not primarily the result of frustrated drive motivation taking the forms of aggressive or libidinal strivings often manifested in unconscious fantasy life. Moreover, attachment need became conceptualized by Bowlby as of lifelong duration, rather than being a phase-specific issue, which in normal development or in the clinical setting is either outgrown or analyzed away, leaving the individual separate and independent. Separateness and independence, free from attachment need, are thus not goals either of normal development or of the treatment situation. Instead, Bowlby viewed optimal attachment as "the secure base" from which the child can then explore his or her world, attaining in this way that quality described by others as autonomy, but always, for Bowlby, existing within a secure attachment system, a quality more akin to interdependence than either independence or autonomy.

Moreover, the familiar motivations so central to classical analysis, libido and aggression, were replaced in Bowlby's system. Bowlby

(1988) came to conceptualize five biologically rooted types of behavior that include, in addition to attachment behavior, exploratory behavior, parenting behavior, sexual behavior, and eating behavior. He noted that his theoretical approach offered a contrast to traditional classical theory: The five biologically rooted motives Bowlby himself identifies—attachment, exploration, parenting, sexuality, and eating—are all treated in classical theory as varying expressions of the traditional dual drives, libido and aggression. Furthermore, aggression is not included in any way as a primary motivation by Bowlby. Rather, aggression is conceptualized as a reactive response to, for example, separation, inadequate attachment, or trauma.

Bowlby (1988) conceptualized these five motivations, instead of the two recognized in classical theory, because each of the five motives serves a distinctive biological function. The functions include protection (attachment), knowledge of the environment (exploration), nurturance (parenting), reproduction (sexual), and nutrition (eating). Moreover, factors that influence the development of each of these motivational behaviors, or systems, can be delineated, and by keeping the systems separate, one can study how they are similar, how they differ, and how they overlap. For example, the child's clinging is born of a motivational origin (attachment) distinct from the parent's caretaking (parenting) behavior. Thus, Bowlby's distinction between the motives of parenting and attachment permits one to conclude that there is a meaningful difference between the parent's attachment to the child and the parent's parenting of that child.

Turning to the clinical situation, Bowlby (1988), addressing the tasks of the therapist, says: "A therapist applying attachment theory sees his role as being one of providing the conditions in which his patient can explore his representational models of himself and his attachment figures with a view to reappraising and restructuring them in the light of the new understanding he acquires and the new experiences he has in the therapeutic relationship" (p. 138). Bowlby then describes the therapist's role, which includes, along with the more expectable explorations of current, past, and transference relationships, the provision for the patient of a secure base from which to explore the painful aspects of his life, "many of which he finds it difficult or perhaps impossible to think about and reconsider without a trusted companion to provide support, encouragement, sympathy, and, on occasion, guidance" (p. 138). At the end of his life, Bowlby, looking back over his lifetime of study and clinical work, notes the two essentials that most impressed him: that attachment is a lifelong experience and need, and that real events have the greatest significance in development and in pathology.

Bowlby defines attachment as a system in which both members of the dyad are vitally affected, each playing a reciprocal role in the evolution and maintenance of the attachment patterns that form between them. Here Bowlby's concept of the importance of both attachment and parenting as separate and distinct primary biological motives inherent in the individual takes the form of particular patterns of both attachment behavior and parenting behavior, which emerge and become elaborated through the mutual influence arising within the parent–child system. In his clinical work, Bowlby focused on the patient's attachment needs. He sought, in therapy, to maintain the patient's already existing secure working models of attachment patterns, to modify pathological working models, and to create new, secure, and more adaptive working models.

FURTHER ELABORATIONS
OF ATTACHMENT THEORY

Mary Ainsworth, working within Bowlby's framework, expanded upon his attachment theory. Using a unique experimental design she devised with her collaborators, termed the Strange Situation (Ainsworth, 1982), she identified three categories of mother–infant attachment patterns and their corresponding parenting patterns. A fourth category was added through the work of Main and Solomon (1986, 1990), as a pattern was identified by them to contain and describe a previously difficult-to-classify group of mother–infant pairs. Following this work, Main and Hesse (1992) explored mother–infant attachment interactions within the context of the home so that the ongoing, day-by-day configurations composed of infant attachment patterns and corresponding parent parenting patterns could be extended beyond the Strange Situation and into everyday life.

The Strange Situation may be described as follows: The child at about a year of age plays in an unfamiliar room, first with the mother present, then with the mother absent (she leaves for a short while), and finally with the mother having returned. Three categories of response were noted by Ainsworth (1982, 1985): one secure pattern and two insecure patterns. First is the category of *secure attachment* (Category B), in which the infant shows moderate anxiety with the mother gone, but is able to be soothed and reassured by the mother on her return, and is then able to return to play. The infant in this category is assumed to be, as Bowlby (1988) states, "confident that his parent will be available, responsive, and helpful should he encounter adverse or frightening situations. With this assurance, he is bold in his explorations of the world. This pattern is promoted by a parent, in the early years, especially by mother, being readily available, sensitive to her child's signals, and lovingly responsive when he seeks protection and/or comfort" (p. 124). So we see here a particular attachment behavior and its corresponding parenting behavior, forming in totality a pattern of attachment and exploration in the infant that is dependent on the secure base provided by the parent. The Strange Situation is a situation designed experimentally to elicit the behaviors the child reveals in separation from and reunion with an important attachment figure, and the behaviors the parent reveals in response to such separations and reunions. The importance of the study, from our perspective, is that the pattern that evolves illustrates a more general pattern of relatedness as well: an ongoing attachment-and-parenting-behavior system characterized by the degree to which the self- and mutual-regulatory patterns within the pair are responsive to the child's attachment needs as opposed to the parent's attachment needs. In the secure attachment, the child is able to explore the world in safety, trusting that the mother will be there without excessive concern about the mother's whereabouts and responsiveness. The mother, in turn, can enjoy the child's explorations without needing to be the center of the child's concern and can then be available when the child returns for more focused maternal parenting responsiveness.

A second category of behavior noted in the Strange Situation, one of the insecure attachment patterns, is termed *anxious resistant (ambivalent) attachment* (Category C), wherein the child is anxious, alternately clinging and rejecting of affection, and the parent is only intermittently emotionally available. As an aside, the description of the child's behavior in this category of attachment is reminiscent of what Mahler (Mahler, Pine, & Bergman, 1975) conceptualized, erroneously we believe, as the rapprochement subphase of separation–individuation, an aspect of normal development to be observed in all children in interaction with their caregivers in the age range of 18–24 months. From our perspective, which was derived from a close, detailed study of Mahler's complete published works, the small, self-selected group of families on which Mahler based her studies was skewed to the pathological (E. Shane & Shane, 1984; Lyons-Ruth

1992). We see this as a testament to the overwhelming importance of continually validating and replicating the experimental studies on which psychoanalytic theories are ostensibly based, and to the need for continually rectifying their findings and conclusions on the basis of new and renewed studies. This latter, more scientifically open-minded approach has been followed in studies on attachment.

In Ainsworth's (1985) description of Category C, the child is described as constantly preoccupied with the parent's whereabouts and responsiveness, with expressions of attachment need being heightened by the parent's only intermittent presence and ability to meet the child's attachment needs. Within the Strange Situation, the child exhibits separation anxiety when the parent leaves and does not comfortably or readily explore the world in the parent's absence. Upon the parent's return, the child alternately clings to and rejects the parent and, above all, cannot be soothed by the parent.

The third category of attachment, also an insecure pattern, is *anxious avoidant attachment* (Category A), wherein the child appears to have no firm expectations of response to his attachment needs, and the parent has repeatedly rebuffed the child's approaches. The child then develops a strategy of keeping all of his or her focused attention away from the parent in order to allow the parent the space he or she apparently requires. It is speculated that the child in this way achieves the greatest physical proximity possible; that is, what is tolerable to the parent. In the Strange Situation, these children explore in an obligatory way, a way postulated to be defensive, apparently noting neither the parent's absence nor the parent's return. Bowlby (1988) notes that "when . . . such an individual attempts to live his life without the love and support of others, he tries to become emotionally self sufficient and may later be diagnosed as narcissistic or as having a false self of the type described by Winnicott" (pp. 124–125).

As we indicated above, in the early investigations by Ainsworth, she discovered that some infants did not fall into any of the three categories of attachment, exhibiting instead, on their reunion with the parent in the Strange Situation, disorganized behaviors such as "freezing," dazed appearance, sudden startle, or playing dead, these reactions alternating with what looked like secure attachment behaviors. It took the further work of Main and Solomon (1986) to identify this aberrant group as an insecure category of its own, which they labeled *disorganized attachment* (Category D). Attachment behaviors in this category were correlated with parents who were abusive, psychotic, or suffering from unresolved losses of their own. It was speculated that the children who fell into this category had achieved no consistently effective strategy to manage separation from the parent and to restore connection with him or her.

Main and Solomon (1986) noted that in all categories of attachment, it was in response to the parent's signal that an infant assumed a given stance in relation to separation from the parent, with the aim of achieving the closest proximity to the attachment figure that the attachment figure could allow. This finding demonstrates the importance of universal attachment strivings in all individuals; the quality of attachment organized in the child is a function of the mutually influencing, parent–child dyad.

It is important to note in this regard that the child may form a different pattern of attachment with each parent, and with any other important caregiver. Again, the operative principle would seem to be that the attachment pattern of the child with a particular parent represents the most secure, closest proximity safely attained by the child and permitted by the parent in that dyad. Thus the child may have more than one attachment pattern to draw on in the course of his or her lifetime of relating to others. Moreover, and of great significance to clinical work, new attachment patterns may be formed with new people coming into the individual's emotional world, an aspect of the positive new experience available with the analyst in our trajectory of developmental progression.

As a final example of the evolution of attachment theory, it has been demonstrated in longitudinal studies covering over two decades (e.g., Sroufe, 1996) that the four categories of attachment pattern identified by Ainsworth (1985) and elaborated by Main and colleagues (Main & Hesse, 1992; Main & Solomon, 1986), can be viewed as persisting in many cases into later childhood, adolescence, and early adulthood. Furthermore, the category of attachment experience in the individual may in some cases persist throughout the life cycle of that individual, though time has not allowed confirmation of this latter hypothesis. We draw extensively on Sroufe's studies in Chapter 3.

CONTRIBUTIONS FROM BOWLBY
AND KOHUT: A BEGINNING INTEGRATION

We have presented this review of attachment theory beginning with Bowlby and elaborated by his followers in order to illustrate the enduring theoretical and clinical contributions of this model to our perspective. We will now identify eight assumptions distilled from attachment theory and integrated, where applicable, with assumptions distilled from self psychology, all of which we include and extend in our own approach.

The first assumption concerns the importance of real life experience as opposed to internal conflict and fantasy elaboration in the development of the individual. Here we accept the emphasis both Bowlby and Kohut placed on lived experience. In addition we note that the defensive self-protections and the creative elaborations of the individual so central in psychoanalytic thought are themselves influenced by or are responses to lived experience, so that some understanding of the individual's lived experience is necessary to comprehend fully these self-protections and creative elaborations in the formation and development of the self.

Second, Bowlby (1969) identifies attachment as a motivation separate and distinct from other motivations. In our approach, too, attachment is a separate motivation. However, we contend that the power and specific role of attachment are better understood as connected to the development of the self. *In our system, the consolidation of the self and the consolidation of the attachment tie to the other become important and intertwined developmental goals in psychoanalysis.* Hence, Bowlby's attachment motivation in the context of a secure base, and Kohut's focus on the centrality of the concept of self as organizer of development, both become elements in a larger system in which the development of self and of the tie to a significant other are inextricably interconnected.

A third assumption we draw from Bowlby's (1988) theory concerns the distinction he makes between the parent's connection to the child and the child's connection to the parent. In the development of a secure base, ideally, the parent parents and the child attaches. This formulation improves and particularizes what is too often confused and generalized in self psychology, when selfobject functions are attributed too broadly to both the parent and the child, or, by analogy, to both the analyst and the patient, in a fashion that is almost symmetrical, though the tilt in the relationship in favor of the patient is, of course, always acknowledged. Something quite valuable, from our perspective, is added, however, when the differences in function are delineated. It is important to note that reverse attachment in the parent–child relationship, that is, the parent using the child for his or her own attachment needs, is distinct from normal, healthy parenting, wherein the attachment tie is not reversed. In self psychology, this theoretical distinction between attachment and parenting does not exist, so that the child's serving selfobject functions for the parent becomes the normal, healthy obverse of the parent's serving selfobject functions for the child, with pathology being defined in terms of excess, that is, an excess utilization of the child for the parent's own selfobject needs (M. Shane & Shane, 1989). Thus, Bowlby's unique delineation and distinction of motives between attachment and parenting provides something that is missing from self psychology.

Fourth, the need for attachment is considered lifelong in Bowlby's framework, just as is the need for selfobject responsiveness in Kohut's framework. Both these models attest to the importance of the self's need for intimate connection with the other. In our model, we distinguish the nature of that intimate tie as either the self in connection with a self-transforming other or as the self in connection with an interpersonal-sharing other, and in addition, we conceptualize both of these intimate attachments as a part of the system "self" and the system "selfother." These concepts will be elaborated in the following chapter.

Fifth, Bowlby contends that separation, independence, and autonomy, as distinct from attachment need, are not legitimate goals in either development or the treatment situation. Instead, what is required in both development and treatment is an ongoing secure base from which autonomy and independence can be seen to derive and on which these capacities can continue to exist. This perspective is consistent with Kohut's contention that separation and independence are inadequate or erroneous as goals in both development and psychoanalytic outcome, and whose concept of the self–selfobject matrix clearly implies interdependence. In our model, too, neither independence nor autonomy are seen as obligatory goals of psychoanalytic treatment whereas attachment and interdependence clearly are.

Sixth, Bowlby (1988) identified five biologically rooted types of motivated behavior: attachment, exploration, parenting, sexuality, and eating. These motivations are similar to the five motivational-functional systems identified later by Lichtenberg (1989), with Lichtenberg repeating, modifying, and elaborating them. Lichtenberg, like Bowlby, sees affiliation as an extension of the attachment motive. He adds assertion to the exploratory motive and sensuality to the sexual motive. Finally, he broadens the category of eating into a general regulation of physiological need. Lichtenberg does not, however, include parenting as a fundamental, biologically based motive, as Bowlby does. Moreover, Lichtenberg adds an aversive motivational system to his list of biologically rooted types of behavior, carrying with it aggressive affect. This last system, in our view, stands in marked contrast to the other four. Ideally, the affect inherent in the aversive system is reduced to a signal function, whereas, in contrast, the affects that accompany the other motivational systems are enhanced, serving as they do developmental selfobject needs for the self.

In contrast to Lichtenberg, and in agreement with Bowlby, we believe that parenting is a significant motive, biologically based and clinically relevant, as we indicated earlier, and as we will further demonstrate shortly. This motive was prefigured long ago by Benedek (1959) when she explicated parenthood as a developmental phase and process. Further, we agree with Bowlby that aversion is not best thought of as a primary motivational system, preferring to see it as both Bowlby and Kohut do, that is, as secondarily reactive to separation, attachment failure, trauma, or any other unfulfilled need state. Moreover, we do not view motivational systems in general as the prime organizers of the clinical moment, as do Lichtenberg and colleagues (Lichtenberg et al., 1992). From our perspective there is no single central organizer of the clinical moment. In addition to many other elements to be identified subsequently, we view the state of the self, the state of the tie to the other, and the establishment of a secure base, as well as, at times, what is motivationally active, as all being essential in assessing the psychoanalytic situation.

In conclusion regarding our sixth assumption, we separate ourselves from Kohut and Bowlby, as well as Lichtenberg and his group, in that we do not conceptualize everything as motivated; we hold that some things just *are*. To illustrate, the brain is organized by and functions to organize experience—this is not motivated behavior, but is an "is" of behavior. More clinically central, the patient's way of organizing the analyst and himself or herself in the intersubjective–interpersonal interaction is not necessarily motivated, but again, may be an "is" of that patient's pattern of organization. For example, the patient who rarely or never looks at the analyst when entering the consultation room may be demonstrating a family-related procedural learning style, nonconscious and without motivational meaning or intention. Finally, aspects of the very gradient of development in the direction of more complexity in organization is not motivated; rather, it is a given of the self (mindbrainbody) that the individual develops to the highest level of organization potentially possible.

The seventh assumption we draw from Bowlby has to do with the role of the therapist. Bowlby (1988) sees the therapist as providing the conditions in which the patient is helped to explore representational models from past and present, restructuring them through understanding and through attempts to establish new, secure working (representational) models. Moreover, Bowlby perceives the therapist, ideally, as a trusted companion who provides support, encouragement, sympathy, and guidance to the patient in these explorations. Bowlby, like Kohut, elaborates positive elements in the treatment situation: Kohut discerns new transferences, which we conceptualize as essentially positive, so that the experiences he delineates of being mirrored, of being allowed to idealize, and of being given a sense of shared humanity are provided the maximal opportunity to emerge within the analytic situation, and stem from the patient's lived experience of unmet selfobject needs. Bowlby devises a system wherein new attachment patterns can emerge with the analyst, who provides, through support, encouragement, and sympathy, a secure base for new explorations in the world. Both focus, then, on security, safety, and predictability in a new relational experience. We accept these ideas from Bowlby as well as from Kohut as basic to our model, with, of course, our clarifications, emendations, and elaborations inherent in the dimensions of relatedness, the relational configurations, the trajectory of developmental progression, and the positive new experience described here and in subsequent chapters.

As an eighth assumption, Bowlby (1988) introduces, as we indicate above, the motives of attachment and parenting. His followers elaborate four basic patterns of bidirectional, mutually influenced attachment behavior and associated parenting behavior in the parent–child unit. In only one of these, the Category B secure attachment pattern, is there an appropriately balanced parent–child relationship, with the child manifesting a predominant pattern of attachment behavior in connection with a parent manifesting a predominant pattern of parenting behavior. In the other three categories of attachment, the insecure attachment categories, there is apparent, from our perspective, a traumatically inverted pattern wherein the child appears to parent the parent but, in fact, on more detailed examination, is actually preoccupied with the parent in ways that interfere with the child's self- and self-with-other consolidation. This last represents our own view of trauma, in which we distinguish ourselves from attachment theorists in general, who see at least two of these three alternative categories of insecure attachment as reasonably adaptive to the circumstances that pertain. Although we do not disagree that these modes of attachment were adaptive in the past, nevertheless they were, from the beginning, instances of trauma, that is, of traumatic attachment in which the child accommodates to the unempathic, poorly responsive, or unresponsive milieu. In addition, although these modes of attachment were adaptive in the past, they do not serve the individual as well as a secure attachment does in the present. This understanding is similar to Brandchaft's (1994) concept of pathological accommodation; however, as we indicated earlier, we prefer to conceptualize as traumatic rather than as pathological such inverted attachment patterns wherein the child's accommodation to the requirements of the parents subvert the child's developmental needs, based on our belief that these responses coming from the child constituted the most adaptive possible at the time, serving self-protective functions.

These ideas have important implications for our developmental systems self psychology approach. As we have indicated, we conceptualize healthy development as the attainment of a consolidated self and a consolidated tie to an intimate other, both of which attainments are consistent with secure attachment experience, and we conceptualize as trauma those outcomes to the self that derive from constitutional and environmental failure, whether with actively abusive and destructive parents, or with absent, neglectful, depressed, or abandoning ones. In our view, such a parental surround contributes to the creation of the categories of insecure attachment that attachment researchers have delineated. These traumatic parenting patterns are most often transgenerational, passed on unconsciously, nonconsciously, and procedurally from the insecure parent of one generation to his or her child in the next. Just as the attachment pattern achieved by the child represents the best and most adaptive self-protective strategy available at the time, so, too, the attachment pattern made available by the parent to the child often represents the best that the parent could do. Moreover, from our perspective, psychoanalytic treatment concerns a change in self- and self-with-other pattern from a traumatized self in connection with a traumatogenic other, to a new, consolidated self in a consolidated tie to a new other, one who serves as a secure base for the future. That is, the secure attachment established in an analytic relationship can serve the dual function of creating both a healthier self and a healthier capacity to parent an other, breaking the transgenerational transmission of insecure parent–child attachment patterns.

Finally, this eighth assumption taken from Bowlby has significant implications for the analyst–patient relationship, in that the analyst assumes, at times, a role analogous to the parent who parents (M. Shane, 1980). The point Bowlby makes, as we indicated earlier, is that this parenting role is different from the attachment role of the child, a distinction that one can analogize to the analyst–patient relationship. Where these roles are confused—where, that is, the therapist uses the patient for his or her own attachment needs instead of providing parenting-like responses, with the attendant satisfactions for both in the dyad—there is danger of creating an inverted analyst–patient attachment relationship akin to the inverted parent–child attachment relationship, with the potential for inflicting or reinflicting trauma on the patient.

DEVELOPMENTAL SYSTEMS SELF PSYCHOLOGY: A NONLINEAR DYNAMIC SYSTEMS INTEGRATION

Thus far we have examined in this chapter two important theories, each of which has contributed major ideas to psychoanalytic thought, and more pertinent here, to our model of developmental systems self psychology. One of these theories, Kohut's self psychology, is essentially a one-person psychology wherein the other serves primarily selfobject functions as a constituent of the self. Here the focus is on the role of that self as organizer of experience, both in development and in the clinical situation. The second of these theories, Bowlby's attachment model, is essentially a two-person psychology wherein self and other are intertwined in an attachment system. Here the focus is on the nature of the interactional patterns that serve to sustain a secure base for the individual, providing for that individual the maximum of proximity accessible in the particular dyad, both in development and in the clinical situation. The divergence of perspectives between these two theories is obvious, one functioning to illustrate the role of self as prime organizer of development, with a cohesive self being the developmental goal; the other functioning to illustrate the role of the secure base as prime organizer of development, with a secure attachment being the developmental goal.

Nonlinear dynamic systems facilitates an integration of these two differing perspectives, bringing them together to help form our model, a developmental nonlinear systems self psychology model that encompasses both these strands, as well as a third strand constituted from findings of developmental systems research and brain research. We are helped in our integrative efforts by the research findings and theoretical conclusions of a number of contributors. These include Peter Fonagy and his colleagues (Fonagy, Steele, & Steele, 1991; Fonagy, Steele, Steele, Moran, & Higgith, 1991), who demonstrate the connection between the establishment of a secure base and the development in the individual of self-reflective awareness, thereby connecting development of self and attachment to the other. We are also helped by Main and Goldwyn (1985), whose studies on narrative formation illustrate the interrelatedness between secure attachment and the capacity to narrate a coherent self-history. Further assistance in our integrative efforts is offered by the findings and theoretical conclusions of other infant researchers, beginning with Louis Sander (1962, 1964), who brought the concept of contingency into the developmental literature, particularizing what constitutes a secure base for the infant, and offering a route to the connection between self-consolidation and consolidation of the tie to the other. Among the many studies conducted in the newborn nursery that illustrate the role of contingent responsiveness in the enhancement of optimal self- and mutual regulation, Sander explored the role of feeding in the development of sleep–wake cycles in the neonate. He discovered that by following the infant's need for feeding (i.e., feeding on demand, as opposed to feeding on schedule), there was a more rapid and successful translation of sleep–wake cycles into a correspondence with night and day, illustrating that contingent responsiveness is correlated with optimal self- and mutual regulation, a surprising finding to those who had conceptualized that development could be controlled most effectively from the outside.

Sander's initial insight regarding contingent responsiveness and its relation to self-regulation and secure attachment has been borne out through the work of subsequent infant researchers, for example Ainsworth (cited in Karen, 1990), who observed and measured the amount of time the infant is held by the caregiver. She notes that in infants who became categorized as securely attached, it was not the amount of time that the caregiver held the infant that created this secure attachment category designation. In fact, the total time that infants were held in both secure and insecure avoidant attachment categories was essentially the same. Rather, what distinguished the two groups was that the securely attached infant was held more often in response to signals coming from the infant, a contingent responsiveness, whereas the insecure avoidant infant was held when the impulse to hold came from the caregiver herself, a noncontingent responsiveness.

Thus, these studies, along with many more, have contributed to our growing understanding of how, through the use of a systems model, connections can be made and patterns discerned even among the immense complexities that constitute human development. It should be clear that we view the integration of self psychology and attachment theory as essential to our model, allowing us to understand the self as it emerges in relationship with the other, and that the state of that self, whether integrated or fragmented, whether consolidated or unconsolidated, is influenced by the quality of that relatedness. For example, when Fonagy (Fonagy, Steele, & Steele, 1991; Fonagy, Steele, Steele, Moran, & Higgith, 1991) connects the achievement of a secure base with the attainment of self-reflective awareness, when Main and Goldwyn (1985) connect the attainment of a secure connection with the evolving capacity to narrate a coherent self-history, and when Sander (1962) connects contingent responsiveness in the surround to the enhancement of optimal self- and mutual regulation, it is the understanding of these complex interactions as nonlinear dynamic systems manifestations that helps to explain and apply these significant connections in our clinical work with patients of all ages.

Thus these nonlinear independent and interdependent elements mutually and persistently influence one another in a fashion that is relatively unpredictable, and yet the parent–child system (and, by analogy, the analyst–patient system) becomes self-organizing, patterned at certain points in the interaction, so that there are relatively predictable aspects as well. That is, referring to the concepts mentioned above, the elements of a secure base, self- and mutual regulation, reflective self-awareness, a coherent self-narrative formation, and a contingent response are linked as complex independent and interdependent elements in the developmental (and analytic) system, with the concomitant occurrence of secure attachment and self-consolidation emerging with some predictability as global patterns.

We are convinced that it is only through the application of a nonlinear dynamic systems perspective that one can at least approach this immense complexity in the effort to conceptualize and integrate these findings from related disciplines into a single model of psychoanalysis, still leaving room for further expansion as scientific, clinical, and theoretical advances occur in the contemporary biopsychosocial field.

Simply put, our definition of a nonlinear dynamic system is any system composed of three or more independent and interdependent elements that, in an ongoing way, mutually influence one another in a fashion that is relatively unpredictable, and yet, the system becomes self-organizing (patterned) at certain points in the interaction so that there is a relatively predictable aspect in the nonlinear system. A good example drawn from the psychoanalytic situation is the concept of transference as defined in our model, that is, the old self with old other, patient–analyst relational configuration. In the psychoanalytic situation, one can predict with relative certainty, that at some point in the course of the treatment, a pattern will emerge (self-organize) in the relationship established between patient and analyst in which both can agree that the patient is experiencing and interacting with the analyst as if that analyst were a significant figure from the patient's past. But one can never predict even with relative certainty when in the analysis this pattern will emerge and, more importantly, what form this patterned relationship from the past will take. Thus, transference represents a nonlinear aspect of treatment, the nature of which cannot be predicted, but the occurrence of which nevertheless becomes a relatively predictable feature in that treatment. Linearity, on the other hand, refers to predictable, cause-and-effect relationships. It is our contention, then, that such linearity only rarely applies to the psychoanalytic situation; that is, relatedness only rarely can be best understood in cause-and-effect terms, but nevertheless some linearities can be identified. There is an absolutely predictable cause-and-effect connection between failure to eat and weight loss, a connection strongly felt by every clinician who attempts to treat the anorexic patient.

At this juncture we will use the currently recognized varieties of self psychology to illustrate the nonlinear systems nature that we find inherent and focal in all contemporary psychoanalytic models. In contrast to more contemporary theories, what had characterized Freudian thinking was the essential linear emphasis inherent in that model. That is, the predominant focus is on the theory-based predictability and the retrospectively reconstructed cause-and-effect relationships, in the clinical situation and in development, made detectable through the analytic method. An obvious example is the concept of universally present dual drive derivatives (e.g., Brenner, 1982), which concept contends that there is an underlying and specific drive causality to any mentation, and furthermore, that where one drive derivative is clinically manifest, it is conceptualized as predictable and inevitable that that drive is only the surface manifestation, that is, one side of the ambivalent duality always expected to be present. Where there is overt love in the transference relationship, for example, there is also underlying, defended-against hate in that transference relationship, which must be eventually confronted, uncovered, and interpreted by the analyst for an analytic process to be said to occur; by the same token, where there is overt hate, there is also underlying, defended-against love that similarly must eventually be confronted, uncovered, and interpreted. This is an instance of a singular cause-and-effect relationship that defines this model of analysis as strongly directed toward linear causality. Freud's model of phases of development, too, is based on linear causality, wherein one phase is inevitably linked to another in progressive and regressive fashion, an innate epigenetic unfolding in predictable sequence. But Esther Thelen and Linda Smith (1994), applying a nonlinear dynamic systems perspective to human behavior and infant development, contend that such single-cause models as are apparent in Freudian thought simply do not account for what one observes in developing organisms, or, we would add, in the developmental aspect inherent in the clinical situation. Thelen and Smith suggest that any innate blueprint is just a shorthand for an unexplained developmental process, a developmental process that is yet to be explicated, but that is presented deceptively as already understood. In other words, what starts out appropriately enough as description of development, however accurate or inaccurate, ends up quite inappropriately as explanation. Freud's *Three Essays on the Theory of Sexuality* (1905)—which outline emotional development in terms of a sequence of phases going from oral, to anal, to phallic, to oedipal, to latency, and finally to adolescence—represent an example of creating the concept of an innate, genetic blueprint for a developmental process that remains nevertheless unexplained.

With the paradigm shift to systems thinking as applied to development, beginning as early as the 1960s in the writings of Sander, we can perceive contemporary models of psychoanalysis as presenting a different explanatory stance, one wherein cause-and-effect linearity is played down, and some efforts are made to include nonlinearity in the system. By looking at self psychology models from this perspective, we can reconcile nonlinear and linear elements in these models through the use of levels of observation, for example, the micro and macro levels articulated by Thelen and Smith (1994). In our view, all models of self psychology are at base nonlinear dynamic systems containing components, patterns, expectations, actions, and outcomes, elements that we will highlight. For example, Kohut's (1971, 1977, 1984) self psychology theory contains such components—patterns, expectations, actions, and outcomes—whose interrelations can be identified, with emergent patterns of which some are predictable and some unpredictable. With a patient who has self-pathology and an analyst who is sufficiently knowledgeable about such pathology and knowledgeable as well about how to sustain an empathic, vicariously introspective listening stance, one could reasonably predict on a macro level and occurring over a macro period of time, that a nonlinear analytic process trajectory, encompassing a selfobject transference pattern, will emerge. Given the components of a particular kind of patient and a particular kind of analyst who performs particular kinds of actions, there are reasonably expectable patterns and outcomes. However, the *specific* pattern that emerges in the system, whether mirroring, idealizing, or alter ego, or a selfobject variety of oedipal relatedness, cannot be predicted, nor can the time of emergence of any pattern be anticipated with certainty. This latter is what Thelen and Smith might refer to as messiness on the micro level, as opposed to the pattern that we describe as emergent on the macro level. Kohut's (1977, 1984) concept of the selfobject transference thus represents for us a nonlinear aspect in Kohut's self psychology system.

Another aspect in Kohut's (1977, 1984) theory we recognize is the postulated "inevitability" of disruption and repair in a well-functioning analysis. For Kohut, given an appropriate patient and a competent analyst, the occurrence of disruption and repair is more or less predictable, but how and when this disruption and repair sequence will emerge is not. Both the relatively predictable occurrence of disruption and repair and the relatively unpredictable timing and nature of the disruption and repair, then, are manifestations of nonlinearity in the psychoanalytic system. What the Kohutian self psychological analyst searches for are patterns in disruption and repair, patterns that, as they are repeated, may become more predictable. There are, as we said earlier, identified components, patterns, expectations, actions, and outcomes in Kohut's overall nonlinear self psychology, and the complex and fluctuating interrelations of these elements are elaborated in that theory.

As a second model of self psychology, Stolorow and colleagues (Stolorow, Brandchaft, & Atwood, 1987; Stolorow & Atwood, 1992; Stolorow, 1997), have reconceptualized self psychology from an intersubjective perspective. The concept of the invariant organizing principle as it emerges in the intersubjective context is a component of their system. Stolorow and his colleagues note that the individual patient has a number of invariant patterns or organizing principles, as does the individual analyst, and that in the patient–analyst system, one or another pattern or principle may emerge into the foreground. Thus, they conceptualize as relatively predictable the emergence from the intersubjective matrix of invariant organizing principles, but exactly which invariant organizing principle evolves is relatively unpredictable, dependent at any given time on the interacting subjectivities of the two participants. Moreover, Stolorow (1997) has already identified Thelen and Smith's (1994) nonlinear dynamic systems theory as an apt metaphor for his own intersubjective approach. To quote Stolorow: "The investigation and illumination of these invariant patterns as they reassemble within the analytic system can produce powerful therapeutic effects in liberating the patient's affectivity and strengthening the patient's capacities for affect integration and articulation" (p. 12). He regards such expansion and enrichment of the patient's affective life in the patient–analyst system as central expectations of an analytic process. Furthermore, Stolorow states, in relation to action in his system, "Effective interpretations are perturbations that *disrupt* the repetitive attractor states [that is, stable patterns] dominating the patient–analyst system, freeing its components to reassemble in new ways, establishing the possibility of alternative principles for organizing experience" (1997, p. 11, italics in original). Thus, the invariant organizing principle serves as one example of a component in Stolorow's overall nonlinear dynamic system. Intersubjectivity and the actions of investigation, illumination, and interpretation become ways to establish alternative organizing principles, and to facilitate the desired outcome of liberating the patient's capacities for affect integration and articulation.

A third model of self psychology is motivational systems and affect theory which has been put forward by Lichtenberg (1989) and his colleagues (Lichtenberg et al., 1992). Here the concept of five distinct motivational systems represents significant components. Nonlinearity is found in the unpredictability of exactly which motivational system will come to the foreground of experience during the analysis at any given time. In this model, the analyst ascertains when in the dyadic interaction the patient's exploratory motivational system emerges into ascendance, for it is at that time that the analyst can more directly and productively pursue an interpretive strategy. When other motivations are in the foreground, the analyst strives to meet these motivational needs in a way that leads to a meliorative, positive selfobject experience. It is through the analyst's striving to meet adequately the patient's selfobject needs, as organized by and expressed within the patient's five motivational systems, that analysis can lead to the patient's self-cohesion, the desired outcome in this motivational systems and affect theory model. This is accomplished by means of such actions on the part of the analyst as expansion of the patient's awareness, self-righting, self-regulation, and interpretation.

Another component in this motivational systems perspective is that of the "model scene," which also emerges in a relatively unpredictable fashion in the dyad. A model scene is a significant event in the patient's life that is co-constructed in the analysis. It often involves a parallel between some important interaction from childhood and some more current interaction between patient and analyst. The model scene cannot be planned, or predictably co-constructed or evoked. This is because the model scene is based on the patient's unique attribution of meaning to evolving interactions with the analyst, together with the analyst's unique actions in response, which taken together create the model scene. The dyad together then connect this scene, whenever possible, with the patient's remembered or unconscious previous life experience, this connection being a desired outcome in this system.

In our model of self psychology we are proposing that the nonlinear aspect be *investigated*. Through this exploration, the nonlinearity itself is recognized as a central organizer of the components and patterns in the system, including the clinician's expectations, actions, and anticipated outcomes. The paradoxical nature of this attempt is obvious; a nonlinear dynamic system contains a mixture of emergent and unpredictable, as well as relatively predictable, patterns, creating an inevitable and ongoing dialectic between anticipated and unanticipated outcomes. Nevertheless we make the assumption that identifying the components, patterns, expectations, actions, and outcomes enhances the likelihood of the analyst's effectiveness in doing analysis. We are speaking here both of the unique, idiographic nature of the analytic venture, and of the attempt to create within that analytic venture more lawful, nomothetic aspects as the patient and analyst gain experience with one another over time, and as the analyst gains experience with many patients over time. Like many of our colleagues, we attempt to distill from within the psychoanalytic situation ways of conceptualizing emergent order among the complexities that pertain there, and it is toward this end that we formulated our theory of developmental nonlinear systems self psychology, focused on the centrality of self, of trauma, and of positive new experience.

THE SELF IN DEVELOPMENTAL SYSTEMS SELF PSYCHOLOGY

We define self in our model as the system *mindbrainbody*. This unique understanding of self integrates concepts from the many sources we have already identified, as well as sources we have yet to discuss. Specifically, we are influenced by Edelman's (1992) concept of the embodied mind, an effort that successfully eliminates remnants of the Cartesian duality of mind and body. We are also influenced by the understanding of self-reflection found in the infant research literature of Main and Hesse (1992), Fonagy et al. (Fonagy, Steele, & Steele, 1991; Fonagy, Steele, Steele, Moran, & Higgith, 1991), and Stern (1985). Finally, we are influenced by the research on memory systems found in the work of contributors whom we have not yet identified here, including Grigsby and Hartlaub (1994) and Clyman (1991).

In our approach, body, brain, and mind are viewed as elements in the total nonlinear dynamic system, self. Self is embedded in larger systems: selfother, that is, the self in interrelationship with a significant other; and selfsurround, that is, the self in interrelationship with the broader significant environment. An important aspect of the self in our model is that we extend the system mindbrainbody beyond the subjective, or even the potentially subjective, to include aspects that are incapable of ever achieving self-reflection.

To help us understand these different aspects of self, we turn to Edelman and the neurophysiology of brain function. What follows is discussed more completely and is more fully related to our model later (in Chapter 4), but for now we will say briefly that Edelman (1992) postulates two kinds of consciousness: primary consciousness and higher-order consciousness. Primary consciousness evolves first, both evolutionarily and in development, and involves being mentally aware of things in the world, of having mental images in the present. Here what is perceived and remembered is only connected with previous experience in the moment, existing only in the present and depending for recall in the future on cues currently extant in the immediate surround. No capacity for self-reflection is yet possible. Higher-order consciousness, in contrast, permits a new ability for awareness of an inner life, and an ability to distinguish between ongoing events in the present and events recalled from the past. The remembered present becomes placed in a framework of past, present, and future, with the individual now possessing an inner life capable of modeling a self that has continuity across time. A reflective self and a comprehensible world are rendered possible.

Edelman (1992) thus presents a neurophysiological model of development of the fundamental self-reflective capacities inherent in all human beings. But the particular degree and quality of self-reflective capacity attained by the individual is a function of the environment, that is, of the selfother and the selfsurround systems within which the individual self develops and learns to relate. Main, Fonagy, and Stern, working individually and with colleagues, each address a particular type of self-reflective awareness manifested in the capacity to narrate a coherent life story, a capacity that is also paradigmatically human, but that nevertheless appears to be related to secure attachment and self-consolidation. Thus a capacity for self-reflection is both a neurophysiological potential in the self, and yet still dependent for its effectiveness on the quality of relatedness available to that self in the selfother system.

How lived experience gets encoded is relevant to our understanding of self and development of self-reflective awareness. We are grateful to the contributions of Grigsby and Hartlaub (1994) and Clyman (1991), who have identified and worked with two distinct and important kinds of memory systems: procedural memory and declarative memory. Procedural memory is a form of *nonsymbolic* encoding wherein the memory is repeated by the individual, behaviorally or emotionally, often out of that individual's awareness. In contrast, declarative memory is a form of *symbolic* encoding, wherein the memory is encompassed in verbal or other semiotic form, and may also be out of awareness.

We have introduced in a short space a number of concepts: mindbrainbody, selfother, selfsurround, coherent life narrative, primary consciousness, higher-order consciousness, procedural memory, and declarative memory. The introduction of these concepts allows us to expand upon the aspects of self in our model.

The aspects of the nonlinear self system we formulate include the *reflective* aspect of self, the *prereflective* aspect of self, and the *nonreflective* aspect of self. We define the reflective aspect of self as that aspect which relies on the achievement of higher-order consciousness; of self-reflective capacity; of symbolic, language-mediated declarative memory, and, in terms of self-narrative formation, of capacities arising from and fostered by a secure attachment. We define the prereflective aspect of self as that aspect of self that is not, or not yet, in awareness, but that is potentially capable of coming into awareness, such as, for example, everyday experiences not currently in focus, procedural memories that are accessible to verbal reflection, and lived experiences and creative elaborative and self-protective fantasies that have been defensively repressed, dissociated, or otherwise sequestered, but that can, under certain conditions, be brought into focus. Finally, we define the nonreflective aspects of self as those aspects that are incapable of ever achieving self-reflection such as, for example, muscular coordination, involuntary muscular control of emotional expression, hormonal levels, synaptic transmission, cerebral blood flow, and cerebellar activity, that is, elements in the self that can never be directly experienced, but, and this is a crucial point, that may vitally affect the self and the self in relation to others. Also included are clinically important procedural memory encodings that are permanently out of conscious awareness, but that nevertheless similarly affect feelings, behavior, and interactions with others.

As an example of one type of nonreflective aspect of self, we can refer to the work of Charles Darwin as it is discussed in Antonio Damasio's (1994) book, *Descartes' Error*, in terms of involuntary muscular control of emotional expression and its role in communication:

> The difference between facial expressions of genuine and make believe emotions was first noted by Charles Darwin . . . in 1872. Darwin was aware of observations made a decade earlier by Guillaume-Benjamin Duchenne about the musculature involved in smiling and the type of control needed to move that musculature. Duchenne determined that a smile of real joy required the combined involuntary contraction of two muscles, the zygomatic major and the orbicularis oculi. He discovered further that the latter muscle could be moved only involuntarily; there was no way of activating it willfully. The involuntary activators of the orbicularis oculi, as Duchenne put it, were "the sweet emotions of the soul." As for the zygomatic major, it can be activated both involuntarily and by our will, and is thus the proper avenue for smiles of politeness. (p. 142)

We quote this illuminating commentary from Damasio (1994) to demonstrate what we intend to convey by expanding our concept of self from subjective experience to that of encompassing the totality of the mindbrainbody as nonlinear dynamic system. We hope to make clear, then, that self is more than subjective self, encompassing the nonsubjective and nonconscious as well, and that communication between self and other is significantly affected by bodily based expression. The clinical significance is obvious and carries with it profound implications. We believe, further, that the example explains the interesting finding drawn from Stern's (1995) work that infants can detect false from genuine expression of emotion. They can distinguish between sham anger and anger, and sham smiles and smiles. Further, Stern noted that babies can detect the depressed mothers' pretense of pleasure from the feelings that lie behind the mothers' attempts at communicating joy, and that such babies themselves display a false smile similar to the mothers'. It is possible to connect the baby's capacity to detect the mother's real feelings to the discovery of Duchenne—that the musculature around both the depressed mother's and her baby's eyes remains fixed and inactivated as the lower half of the facial musculature moves into the familiar polite smile expression.

In one clinical case, we can see how a nonreflective aspect of the analyst affected her patient's relationship with her. The patient was a physical therapist highly knowledgeable about and sensitive to gait disturbances. One day in the context of the patient's attempting to understand her persistent mistrust of her analyst, the patient noted spontaneously that the analyst seemed to be unsteady on her feet. The patient's revelation came as a total surprise to her analyst. The analyst had never herself been aware of her own unsteadiness, and she could barely perceive it even when brought to her attention. Exploring the meanings of this perception to the patient opened a floodgate of connections to the patient's sense of her analyst as an unreliable, unpredictable, undependable person, contextualizing these percep-tions within the patient's awareness of her analyst's subtle physical defect. The unsteadiness had remained outside of the analyst's aware-ness until it was clarified for her by the patient, at which time the meanings could be investigated and specific light shed on the more pervasive problem of the patient's mistrust of her analyst.

To continue our discussion of the self, we distinguish in our perspective as well between an *integrated* self state and an *unintegrated* self state, and between a *consolidated* self state and an *unconsolidated* self state. An integrated self encompasses attributes marked by agency, coherence, affectivity, and historicity (Stern, 1985). An unintegrated self lacks these attributes to a significant degree. Here self states are rendered discontinuous, by, for example, the self-protective strategy of dissociation, so that agency, coherence, affectivity, and historicity are fractured and disrupted amongst self states. Consolidation of the self includes the following qualities: First, the qualities that describe an integrated self state, that is, agency, coherence, affectivity, and historicity; second, an intersubjective capacity, that is, a capacity to understand and appreciate that the other has a mind that can be shared; third, a sense of and conviction about what is real; fourth, creative self-elaborative strategies, that is, the ability to use fantasy, play, and thought to improve upon and enrich one's life so that pleasure can be both self-generated and shared with another; fifth, adaptive self-protective strategies, that is, the ability to revise self-protective defenses originally constructed as most adaptive to past traumatic life circumstances so that the defenses now reflect more current, less traumatic life circumstances; sixth, self-reflective capacities, which include the achievement of a coherent life narrative, and an ability to distinguish among past and present in terms of the relative influence of each on self and other; seventh, the achievement of a secure attachment, a consolidation of the intimate tie to the other. In contrast, the nonconsolidated self state, although achieving the attributes of integration, may lack flexibility in any or all of the above-listed capacities pertaining to a consolidated self state.

SELF, MOTIVATION, AND DEVELOPMENTAL NONLINEAR DYNAMIC SYSTEMS SELF PSYCHOLOGY

Earlier we discussed the role of self as a prime organizer of development, with a cohesive self being perceived as the goal in development (as put forward by Kohut and his followers), along with the role of the secure base as a prime organizer of development, with secure attachment being perceived as the goal in development (as put forward by Bowlby and his followers). At this point we turn to our third strand, developmental systems research and brain research (as put forward by Edelman, 1992, and Thelen & Smith, 1994), to introduce the developmental dynamic systems self psychology perspective on motivation and the self.

Edelman (1992) postulates that self-organization is categorized and continuously recategorized on basic values, which are genetically inborn as well as emergent over time, based on lived experience within the systems we identify as self, selfother, and selfsurround. We conceptualize that these values then coalesce and develop in a nonlinear fashion into the larger patterns of action and motivation.

What are these basic values, these biases, discoverable both in Edelman's conceptual understanding and that of Thelen and Smith?

Edelman (1992) constructed a series of robots in order to demonstrate a real-life working model illustrating his view of mind–brain functioning. He built into each robot specific values upon which the robot's experience with the surround was continuously categorized and recategorized. The values built in were kept simple; for example, light is better than no light and contact is better than no contact. Edelman and Tononi (personal communication, 1995) indicated that it is not yet known how complex these values are in the neonate and how predictably these values progress into motivational systems. It is known that values do include a repertoire of around 100 inborn reflexes, including such value-based behaviors as rooting, sucking, startle, reaching, and grasping. Edelman and Tononi indicated as well that there may be more complex values inherent in earliest life, including, for example, attachment per se, but that as of now, such inclusion of complexity in developmental theory is not possible. There is just not enough known about how values organize and reorganize neuronal nets and brain maps in the growing child.

Thelen and Smith (1994), too, believe that a plausible developmental scenario for the human infant can be created upon equally simple values, which organize for the infant the as-yet-unlabeled surround. According to these authors, the values might be something like the infant's perceptual scan of the environment with biases toward edges, toward movement, toward the human voice, toward warmth, or toward touch, and, further, that such discoveries by the infant in the surround can initiate in him or her a cascade of progressive development.

We speculate that the infant, having begun with a relatively stark set of values, over time, in interaction with the surround, develops the more complex motivations identified by psychoanalytic theorists. These motives, emerging in self-development, may then become *stable configurations* or enduring patterns (attractor states) in the nonlinear dynamic system (see Chapter 5 for a more extended discussion of attractor states and their use in our model). The necessity for conceptualizing some values as inherent was provided by Edelman and Tononi in our conversation (personal communication, 1995). They made the observation that were humans to be initially without values around which organization of experience could take place, the system mind–brain (or, in our model, the system mindbrainbody) would either freeze around a few nonflexible patterns, or would spin out of control into unformulated chaos. Values thus become a necessary orientation or compass for patterning, or, put in terms more familiar to psychoanalysts, motivation serves as a key element for self-development.

Having identified the origins and some of the essential features of our model, we can, in the chapters that follow, discuss the other aspects of our developmental systems self psychology framework.

CHAPTER THREE

The Two Dimensions of Intimacy

In this chapter we elaborate the two dimensions of intimacy in the psychoanalytic situation. These dimensions describe how patient and analyst connect with one another in that setting, with "self" referring to the patient, and "other" referring to the analyst. We term the two dimensions the *self-transforming* dimension and the *interpersonal-sharing* dimension. The self-transforming dimension refers to the intimate relationship between the self (the patient) and the self-transforming other (the analyst); the interpersonal-sharing dimension refers to the intimate relationship between the self (the patient) and the interpersonal-sharing other (the analyst).

We introduced these dimensions in the first two chapters and established how intimacy plays an important role in the movement toward consolidation of the self and consolidation of the tie to the other. We differentiated our concept of the self with self-transforming other from Kohut's (1971, 1977, 1984) concept of the self–selfobject and from Stern's (1985) concept of the self with self-regulating other. We then briefly delineated our concept of the self with interpersonal-sharing other. We want to begin this chapter with a fuller description of the importance to our clinical theory of the interpersonal-sharing dimension of intimacy.

Long before we began to write together, we found as individual practitioners that an interpersonal approach, as opposed to an impersonal approach, was clinically essential in our efforts to understand and to be therapeutically helpful to our patients. The sharing and giving of oneself in relating to the patient constitutes a crucial source of the positive new experience that we seek to establish and provide. It is in this realm in particular that our own contributions clinically and theoretically are most pertinent, then, because it is in this realm in particular that psychoanalysis and psychoanalysts have been most stifled and their intimate voices most muzzled, under the constraints imposed by the prevailing concepts of abstinence, neutrality, fear of gratifying, worry about uncontrollable regression, privileging of frustration, and concern about missing unconscious meanings. As individuals we have had numerous personal and professional experiences with local, national, and international organized psychoanalysis in which we have been told in one way or another that being a warm, caring, and optimistic human being is antithetical to analytic process. This view, however couched, has always conflicted with our experience, in which we combined medical, pediatric, educational, and clinically based psychoanalytic work with infants and children within their families, and then with individuals across the lifespan (e.g., Gales, 1978). This knowledge born of life in many different areas has thoroughly convinced each of us that it is in the human realm of caring and love that any form of meliorative change must take place.

Self psychology offered us a more compatible approach than had classical theory, coming closer to our ideal of serving the human needs of the patient and of taking the patient at face value, that is, valuing the patient's subjective experience, but without overlooking or slighting sequestered or dynamically unconscious problems. In our own clinical experience, then, the selfobject concept has been quite useful both in understanding development and in conceptualizing the analytic situation. Yet this concept did not explain or describe all of the varieties of intimacy that pertain there. Each of us in our own ways has always been convinced that conceptual space must be made for additional and equally important forms of connection, and for comprehending how the patient and analyst each lives with and experiences the other within their connection. First efforts by two of us (e.g., M. Shane, 1991; M. Shane & Shane, 1989, 1993) involved the division of such experience into two dimensions: the selfobject dimension, defined as the patient's perception of the analyst as a function for the self; and the selfother dimension, defined as the patient's perception of the analyst as a person in his or her own right. Our subsequent thinking as a threesome has evolved further in this respect, attempting to capture more fully the essence of the positive human relatedness so essential to the patient's improvement. This value, based though it is largely on our own individual and collective life experiences, has been buttressed significantly by knowledge derived over time from other fields, specifically attachment and infant research and observation, developmental systems research, and brain research.

The dimensions of intimacy we currently recognize, the self-transforming and the interpersonal-sharing, represent heuristic distinctions that separate two clinically relevant ways of self being with other within a positive—that is, development-enhancing—connection, and these dimensions are important in relatedness outside of the clinical setting, as well. Both dimensions of relatedness, self-transforming and interpersonal sharing, then, must be made available to the developing child by the environmental surround, and ideally remain available to the individual throughout the course of life. Moreover, the healthy person even in early childhood partakes in giving and receiving both self-transformative and interpersonal-sharing experiences for and with important others. That said, we want to emphasize strongly that there is a change in the balance between responding to the other's needs for intimacy and receiving from the other experiences of intimacy, with that change being dependent on the age and developmental needs of the individuals in any given dyad. With the child in relation to the parent, it seems obvious that the child's needs for intimacy should remain paramount, and that the child does not provide either self-transforming or interpersonal-sharing experiences for the parent in anything like an equal measure. Where the connection being explored is between two adults, as in friendship, marriage, or collegial connection, for example, there is ideally an equality of provision for each other's self-transforming and interpersonal-sharing needs, though at times one person may require more of each kind of experience than the other person. In the clinical situation, it is the patient's developmental needs that are always foremost. Whether the dimension of intimacy in ascendance in the dyad is transformational or interpersonal depends on how the needs of the patient are conceptualized at that time. The patient with analyst may be thought of as akin to the child with parent in terms of whose needs for intimacy are viewed as most important, and which dimension of intimacy is postulated as emergent at that time.

Intimacy in our framework encompasses the relatedness that develops between patient and analyst based on the patient's beginning sense of trust and confidence in the analyst. When the connection between patient and analyst begins in an old self with new other relational configuration (old–new), or in a new self with new other relational configuration (new–new), some form of intimacy exists from the inception of the analysis because some sense of positive and distinct otherness is present right from the beginning. But when the analyst is perceived as a traumatic other from the past, and the patient perceives himself or herself as the traumatized self from the past—that is, wherein the relational configuration is old–old—intimacy is not and cannot be present. Therefore, in our model intimacy only occurs when the analyst has emerged in the patient's experience from the old self with old other relational configuration sufficiently to be seen as distinct and different from the traumatic other from the patient's past, so that some sense of positive otherness becomes possible. In sum, intimacy in developmental systems self psychology is based in the positive new experience. Once the patient has been helped to move into the present to some extent in relation to the analyst, the forms intimacy takes become increasingly expanded during the course of treatment. Not only do we anticipate that the patient in a well-functioning analysis will be able to relate to the analyst in both dimensions of intimacy, so that there are experiences of both the self-coming-into-being (self-transforming) and the self-coming-into-connection (interpersonal sharing), but also the extent of intimacy in each dimension is broadened, and the emotional life becomes wider and deeper.

Although intimacy is based in positive new experience, we want to be very clear that "positive" does not necessarily mean positive emotions. Indeed, the emotion in the moment constituting a positive new experience may be negative. For example, a young patient, always compliant in her relationships with older people, came into contact with a fragile elderly woman who had had difficulty in negotiating the automatic ticket dispenser in a parking structure. The patient was in a hurry and found herself in a rage. Bolting out of her car, she grabbed the ticket out of the dispenser and threw it into the woman's car. She said contemptuously, "If you are too old to drive, you shouldn't be driving!" Completely cowed and presumably shamed, the woman hurriedly drove off, leaving the patient remorseful, but with a larger sense of mastery and relief. Reluctantly relaying the story to her analyst, the patient noted that though she had behaved meanly to the other driver, and feared her analyst's disapproval, she nevertheless felt victorious. The woman had not died consequent to her actions, an old fear from childhood, and the analyst had not withdrawn. In fact the whole incident led to a broadened capacity to be rageful with her analyst whom, it was discovered, she also saw at times as feeble and fragile. Positive new experience suggests instances in the safety and security of a relational configuration in which intimacy is possible and in which the patient can relay any range of affects, saying what he or she feels, however dysphoric, sad, angry, or attacking the feelings. All feelings are welcomed and accepted as expressions of authentic emotion in the positive new experience.

As another example, a patient cried at an early point in her analysis, feeling isolated, hopeless, and abandoned. She was in an old–old relational configuration that had recaptured her oft-repeated childhood experience of being sent to her room to cry alone. Intimacy was absent in the dyad, and the experience was neither positive nor new. Later in the analysis this same patient began to cry, but this time felt relief and had the expectation that the analyst would express a soothing concern for her state. The same negative affect, then, became in this instance a positive new experience wherein, in an old–new relational configuration moving toward a new–new pattern, the patient could now feel the analyst's presence and comfort, and no longer felt so alone.

Finally, an expression of deep and direct anger with the analyst can represent a positive new experience for the patient, and where that anger is reciprocated and then worked through, it can represent as well an enhancement of interpersonal-sharing intimacy and understanding between the pair. For example, a patient arrived late once again to see his analyst. Coming late had been the subject of some exploration between them, and the analyst commented once again about it. The patient then asserted, "You're really angry with me, aren't you?" The analyst did not feel angry and said so, but acknowledged a mild frustration about the patient's being late so often. The patient then insisted that the analyst was not just frustrated, but in fact was only soft-pedaling the much greater and more profound emotion of rage. The analyst questioned her patient as to why he was so convinced that the analyst felt something other than what the analyst herself was aware of feeling, and the discussion went back and forth in this vein, becoming increasingly heated, with the analyst finally asserting that the patient's insistence that she was enraged, even when the analyst said she was not, was indeed enough to create the very anger in her that the patient had so relentlessly maintained was there to begin with. The analyst's retort seemed to break the tension that had been growing between them, both of them being amused by the paradoxical situation that they had co-created, with the intimacy between them being enhanced by their sharing together negative feelings in a new and positive way.

THE SELF-TRANSFORMING DIMENSION
OF INTIMACY: A DESCRIPTION

In the first dimension of intimacy, the self-transforming dimension, the analyst is experienced by the patient as an other who provides significant functions for the self. These functions include self-regulation, self-affirmation, self-protection, self-expansion, self-delineation, self-cohesion, self-sustenance, and self-state regulation and stabilization. Moreover, self-reflection, the finding of meaning, and the formation of narrative in terms of self-experience are important aspects in this dimension. All of these functions are encompassed within the self-transforming dimension of intimacy, the broad experience of the self coming-into-being potentiated by the relationship with an other.

A patient who suffered from an inability to sleep at night and who was too agitated to remain at home during the day with her children, continually distracted herself by shopping and having nonpleasurable but time-consuming lunches with friends in an unsuccessful effort to self-regulate. She discovered in analysis that so long as she could remember she had felt the fear that she would be overwhelmed by unbearable states of anxiety, that she would black out, be unable to breathe, and just disappear. Although aware of these feelings, she could not reflect on them until she felt safely connected to her analyst. Within the self-transforming connection to her analyst, the patient experienced an intimacy that provided self- and mutual-regulatory experiences for the first time in her life. Her sleep disorder gradually· became manageable and, with it, her ability to feel safe at home when she was alone with her children.

Another patient fell into dissociative states of blankness in the session. When she returned to a more normal state, the analyst was able to tell her what she had just experienced. Eventually the patient could relate to the analyst while in the dissociative state so that the analyst became the bridge between the two states of the patient's self, the analyst becoming in effect a self-state integrator and self-state stabilizer in the self-transforming dimension of intimacy.

This category of intimacy is characterized by a number of specific attributes. Briefly, these attributes include, first, the essentially positive nature of this relatedness. Even when the patient experiences negative or dysphoric affect, the analyst nonetheless still provides a consistent ambience of hope, optimism, and safety. Moreover, this essentially positive ambience is experienced by the analyst as well. What makes the experience positive for the patient, even in the context of negative emotions felt by either or both, as we have just illustrated, is the movement toward a positive self-transformation growing out of the experience, whether that experience has a positive or negative affect tone. And there is always for an analyst some pleasure in an expanded awareness of the patient's self states, even when those self states are angry, hostile, or dismissive. Moreover, there is for the analyst the pleasure that comes from providing a development-enhancing experience for an other, and as well some sense of competence that derives from performing one's professional functions adequately. Incidentally, we conceptualize this pleasure in the analyst as deriving not so much from the patient's providing self-transforming experiences for the analyst's self, but more as deriving from the motivation identified by Bowlby as parenting, and conceptualized by M. Shane (1977) as "analysthood," in analogy with parenthood. In any case, whether the transformational experience arises from positive or negative affective interchange, the indicator is often the patient's self-description in a given exchange referring to "the new me."

To provide an example, a patient told her analyst in exhaustive but emotionless detail of an exercise regime she had subjected herself to over the weekend in order to deal with bodily tensions that had greatly troubled her. The affectless, repetitive account of this regime threatened the analyst with feelings of boredom and inattention. He was only able to remain alert and interested by reminding himself that at least his patient was now able to translate the details of her bodily states into word. He was then able to make a connection to the patient's competitive strivings as a gymnast during her latency. She had suffered at that time from undifferentiated dysphoric affects manifested by painful muscular tension in her legs whenever she did not receive a perfect score from the judges, forcing herself to practice longer and harder in order to deal with this emergent tension that came from not being good enough. She had received no help from her parents throughout her childhood in either recognizing or dealing with her feelings, eventuating in bodily expression rather than verbal expression of unpleasant emotion. As an adult, bodily tension required that she go through that same excessive exercise routine in order to regulate that tension at a manageable level. By getting through the boredom and staying with the patient's feelings, the analyst functioned as a self-transforming other, helping the patient to differentiate more specifically the feeling states that during childhood were unacceptable to her parents. In turn, the analyst was rewarded by the sense of competence that comes from serving as a self-transforming other for his patient, feeling a quiet satisfaction in a job well done, and above all, in having helped his patient to feel better. We want to distinguish in this example the origins of the analyst's pleasure. Here the patient is not conceived of as serving self-transformative functions (or interpersonal-sharing functions) for the analyst, resulting in a pleasurable experience for the analyst. Rather, the analyst's own pleasurable experience derives from serving well and adequately the functions of an analyst, like the parenting pleasure that comes from nurturing a child.

A second emphasis in the self-transforming dimension derives from the ever-present mutual influence and bidirectionality of interaction in the dyad. This is important to note, especially in those cases in which the patient feels such dysphoric affects as hopelessness and despair, or anger and disappointment. Clearly these emotions affect the analyst, requiring a sustained effort on the analyst's part not only to empathize with and understand the patient's dysphoric feelings, but also to communicate another, additional perspective, if only through his or her inner, not directly verbalized, attempts to balance the dysphoria with optimism and hope.

An example of such failure of balance can be taken from an analyst's experience with a patient who repeatedly complained of not ever getting anything of value from her analytic experience. The analyst had in the past struggled to maintain a sanguine attitude, but for whatever unknown reasons, in this session the analyst felt herself giving way to the patient's sense of hopelessness and despair, unwittingly matching the patient's dysphoric tone with her own. Then she helplessly watched as the patient and she herself seemed to sink together into apathy, and she found she was able neither to recover nor to help her patient to recover. What was surprising was the powerful effect on the patient. Heretofore the analyst had believed that her patient was as depressed and hopeless as one could possibly imagine a person to be, but she now witnessed the patient plunging even further into despair, apparently potentiated by resonating with the analyst's nonverbal response. The bidirectional mutual influence inherent in this experience was confirmed. In the session that followed, the patient commented upon the despair she felt because the analyst, too, felt that the patient could not be helped.

This case also illustrates aspects of the third attribute of this dimension of relatedness, namely, the patient's awareness of the other as always being there as an other, even in the self-transforming connection. In this case, the patient was clearly conscious of her analyst and of her analyst's self state. In the self-transforming dimension of intimacy, such awareness of the analyst as a separate person is conceptualized as always present, though the use to which the analyst is put excludes the analyst's subjectivity, motives, intentions, and/or emotions as being important to the patient except insofar as they are experienced by the patient as operating in the service of the patient's own well-being. The analyst in this example was accurately perceived by the patient as the "downtuner" and the "uptuner" of the patient's affects, that is, as a self-regulator of the patient's emotional states.

Finally, a fourth attribute of this dimension of intimacy is that the patient's experience of the self-transforming other is postulated to be a positive new experience, one not based on templates from the past. It is thus in our framework neither a transference manifestation nor a transference-like manifestation.

As a final example, a young woman complained bitterly to her analyst one day about a good friend's slighting her by canceling a small dinner the woman had been planning to celebrate the patient's birthday. The patient, Kathy K., had been depending on the dinner to alleviate her aloneness on that day. The depth of her pain, genuine and understandable, was the center of her focus, and it was only in passing that she noted to her analyst the reason for the cancellation: Her friend was pregnant, having struggled for years to achieve this, and was now at risk of losing her child and was ordered by her physician to remain on bed rest. Kathy could talk about this situation, and note her own reluctance to commiserate with her friend's grief. She said, "I tell her everything about myself, and I always expect her to feel for me, but I cannot hear about or feel for her, and I am not even interested in it."

The patient was able on her own to see the irony of the situation, the lack of symmetry in the relationships she establishes. Yet for this patient, even this limited capacity to know another's perspective, though she was unwilling to address it with her analyst, represents an analytic attainment of self-reflective capacity. Her attainment of enhanced self-reflection grew out of feelings of safety and security facilitated by an extended self-transforming other relationship with her analyst in an old–new configuration; that is, despite the fact that Kathy still felt in old familiar ways, unable to empathize with an other when her own needs went unmet, she was nevertheless able to see her analyst as different from previous caretakers, and was therefore able to experience positively and as new the relationship between them, and to use it effectively for her own self-development.

In this instance, the analyst affirmed Kathy's feelings of loneliness without any attempt to draw attention to or to interpret the patient's self-protective distancing from her own discomfort with her perception of this imbalance she establishes in connections with others. That is, the analyst neither confronted her with her developmental incapacity nor interpreted its origins. Moreover, and directly to the point we are attempting to make here, the analyst did not in any way bring the experience into an interpersonal-sharing dimension of the relationship, revealing, for example, the analyst's own responses at being similarly treated by the patient as a function of the patient's self needs, not valued as a person in her own right. Rather, the analyst took into account the intimacy dimension currently at the forefront of the analysis, the self with self-transforming other pattern. In doing so, the analyst was encouraged by the transforming benefits that this dimension of intimacy was effecting and had already effected in the patient, benefits observable to the analyst by the patient's new capacity to self-reflect, and observable by the patient, as well, in her sense of feeling, as she had put it many times, safe and protected for the first time in her life. This feeling of encouragement the analyst felt in her patient's progress addresses the pleasure she took, the positive new experience for the analyst herself in being able to facilitate her patient's development.

We believe that were the analyst to respond differently, by, perhaps, prematurely introducing, or forcing into the dyad, her own feelings, or were she to interpret the patient's acknowledged discomfort with her asymmetric relationships, as exemplified by the patient's ironic comments about the contrast between herself and her pregnant friend in regard to being able to feel for an other, we imagine that rather than achieving an interpersonal-sharing other intimacy with Kathy, the analyst would probably have disrupted the ongoing, meliorative, positive new self-transforming experience. And in so doing, the analyst might even have provoked an impasse in the analytic relationship. She might have unnecessarily revived past traumatic experiences wherein the patient was required to abandon her own self needs in order to consolidate the tie to the other, accommodating to the analyst's requirements of her. Or, she might have become enraged with the analyst, and then withdrawn in such a way that repair, if possible at all, would require considerable work, and a loss of trust might ensue.

Some might view this approach as inauthentic, a sacrifice of the analyst's own genuine feelings in relation to the patient. An analyst might have introduced more of her own feelings in the interaction described. This analyst might have told Kathy that she had at times felt with Kathy as she imagined Kathy's pregnant friend might have felt, that her own personhood had been ignored or invalidated. In the search for the most "authentic" response, the analyst might have introduced these feelings into an exploration of the birthday party and its cancellation. Our experience is that authentic feelings are complex, not singular, and that to be authentic as an analyst may at times require no more than a maintenance of genuine concern for the transformational experiences required by the patient, regardless of whatever other reactions the analyst might be having. We accept that perhaps Kohut's greatest contribution to our understanding of this dimension of intimacy, his self–selfobject relationship, is that, as analysts, it is a violation of our pact and commitment to the patient to be other than nonmoralistic and accepting, knowing that the patient's feelings, however they may appear from a conventional point of view, should be safely contained and accepted without fear of recrimination or retaliation and, in fact, with a legitimate expectation on the patient's part of helpful, positive responsiveness.

It was in this attitude of Kohut's that a revolutionary change in the treatment of self disorders such as Kathy's was offered, and it is this same attitude that informs our approach in the self-transforming dimension of intimacy. We should note, however, that the question might still arise even in self psychology, is the analyst trying to avoid a disruption and therefore missing an opportunity for a structure-building experience of disruption and repair? We can only respond to that question (which we can imagine coming from our self psychological colleagues) that, in our model, alternative responses are always an option where it is felt that confrontation might subject the patient to a retraumatization experience, an experience, that is, that the patient is as yet unable to reflect upon and hence unable to gain from, and that consolidation of the self can arise just as effectively from responsiveness that allows the patient to go on being in the relationship. We can look for support to Bowlby (1988) and his parenting motivational system. One aspect of parenting is providing a safe and development-enhancing environment for the child, which inevitably includes keeping parts of his or her own experience private.

THE INTERPERSONAL-SHARING DIMENSION OF INTIMACY: A DESCRIPTION

In the self with interpersonal-sharing other dimension of intimacy, the analyst is experienced by the patient in a two-person, bidirectional, mutual influence system as an other whose self, motives, intentions, emotions, and subjectivity are appreciated for their own sake, and not just in relation to the patient's needs. Unlike in the self-transforming dimension, the patient's sense of intimacy in this dimension is based on interpersonal sharing, which includes subjective, intersubjective, and procedural sharing as well as other nonsubjective experiences of self-coming-into-connection-with-other. Interpersonal-sharing intimacy also includes other kinds of connectedness and communication, both known and unknown, in which mutual, shared meaning finding in verbal form has a significant place. Overall, this dimension encompasses an appreciation for the other as having a self of his or her own, the uniqueness of which is of interest to the other. It also encompasses a positive new experience of a shared humanity, a heightened mutuality, affection, liking, and even love exchanged between the two participants in the analytic dyad, not always equally, and above all, not ever without the patient's development maintained as central to the interaction between them. The analyst's experience in this dimension of intimacy is very much like that of the patient's, with the exception that the analyst's central focus remains on the patient's developmental needs. Like the self-transforming dimension, the interpersonal-sharing dimension is not considered to be transference, but is viewed as new, never-before-encountered experience, providing a new template for similar intimacy outside of the analytic relationship. An expanded range of feelings toward the analyst thus becomes possible. This expansion includes the potential not only for hate and other dysphoric emotions where such emotions are genuinely felt, but equally as important, it includes the potential for love, and, moreover, for the many other feelings that may be experienced along the way, such as anger, shame, guilt, depression, anxiety, joy, surprise, pleasure, and sexual excitement.

Psychoanalytic theory has always considered hatred and aggression to be the most crucial and problematic emotions encountered by the analyst. In our model, however, love takes an equally important position. In fact, it appears that love has come to present even more difficulties in the clinical situation than either hatred or aggression. In the contemporary world, the analyst's feelings of hatred—and even at times expressions of hatred, toward the patient are often more acceptable than the analyst's feelings of love, and even at times expressions of love, toward the patient, not to mention feelings and expressions of lust. One reason for this problematic aspect is the increasingly legalistic milieu in which we all live and practice. By keeping in mind the patient's development as the organizing principle for all of the analyst's actions, some of the analyst's constraints in these matters may be reduced, allowing greater freedom, spontaneity, and originality so that actions and emotions may be considered that are truly and justifiably in the patient's best interests, from the analyst's perspective. We will now introduce three clinical vignettes that address love in the analytic relationship, in the interpersonal-sharing other dimension of intimacy.

A patient, secure in a well-established analytic relationship, had a moving exchange with her analyst in which she felt profoundly understood by him as never before, and helped by him to a never-before-achieved self-acceptance. What did that analyst do with the expectant pause that followed after she said to him, for the first time in their relationship, "I love you"? What could that analyst say then to his patient about what he felt in response? And how long did he have to figure this out? From our perspective, he surely could not say nothing in that ensuing silence. Nor in this instance, which we recognize to be an emergent interpersonal-sharing dimension of intimacy in a new self with new other relational configuration, could he have made an interpretation designed ostensibly to promote in his patient even greater insight, but actually, perhaps, designed to gain some time for his own self-reflection. After all, these were new feelings coming from the patient that might legitimately have generated in the analyst counter feelings of surprise and uncertainty. Nevertheless, from our perspective, neither silence nor interpretation nor delay of any kind would have been a properly attuned, optimal response, one that promoted developmental progression. In this context, taking into consideration the concept of dimensions of intimacy, and recognizing in the patient's strong, affective expression a wish for a genuine experience with an interpersonal-sharing other, and, moreover, having truly been with his patient in that meaningful moment, and aware of his own corresponding wish for such an intimate connection, with all that in mind, this analyst felt he could only say, with equal feeling and engagement, "I love you, too."

Now, how can this analyst have done this? He could do this because in today's analytic zeitgeist, and from our perspective, affective responsivity is understood as an important, indeed necessary, dimension of the relationship, the positive new experience between patient and analyst. The analyst's feelings of love, *before* his patient's expression of profound feeling, may not have been deliberately, consciously communicated, and perhaps were not even consciously felt by him, but during the previous highly charged, intimate exchange wherein the patient had felt so completely known, his own emotions were not only aroused, but also, perhaps, communicated on some level, procedurally, nonverbally, through the total self state, which includes such important aspects as behavior, state of arousal, and the curve and contour of temporal feeling shapes (Stern, 1995). In fact, we think that *without* such affective resonance coming from the analyst, communicating his *own* empathic involvement, this patient would not have felt safe or open enough to have professed her heartfelt feelings in the first place. In this sense, the analyst's communication is ongoing and is not even in conscious control. The analyst, then, discloses feelings whether or not he knows it, and often by the same measures that the patient has disclosed to him: *nonverbally*, procedurally and through actions; and *paraverbally*, through the music accompanying the declarative language that the patient employs.

We want to make the point also that in a dimension of intimacy that is characterized by the patient's wish for interpersonal-sharing intimacy, it is important to resonate accurately and responsively with the patient's affective communication. This require a communication that encompasses an authentic affective response of one's own, ideally a communication that affectively matches that of the patient. When the patient in our example says to her analyst, "I love you," then, were her analyst to have responded with something that conveys only his own fondness, for example, "I care very much about you, too," the effect might be to down–tune the patient's genuine and open expression of affection, running the risk of humiliating or, at the least, deflating the patient's self. Were he using another theoretical framework, the analyst in our example might have hesitated to express such strong feelings directly, with the fear that he would be perceived, either by the patient, himself, or the imagined analytic community, as seductive. However, from our perspective, such genuine affect expressed with the intention always of providing for the patient a positive new experience, is salutary in the analytic process.

It would seem appropriate to ask, at this point, what kind of love, or what kinds of love, are being shared in this new, positive moment between self and other in this interpersonal-sharing dimension? Conceptualizing an increased range of motivational possibilities, we postulate that not all love is libidinal, not all love is sexual or erogenous, oral, anal, phallic, genital, and the like. *Nonsexual attachment* is understood to be a significant and powerful experience of mutual love in the analytic setting. Affiliation is important, as well. Caregiving, self-regulatory functions are also infused with love. And we believe, certainly more controversially, that even the analyst's sexual feelings are permissible, and even acceptable to convey to the patient, under certain conditions—that is, only when the patient would benefit from knowing, and only so long as one is not violating either legal restraints, which forbid physical sexual and physical aggressive contact, or one's own contract to put first and foremost the patient's well-being. For example, an elderly, physically handicapped patient asked her analyst if he found her sexually attractive at all. He responded honestly that he did. She found it impossible to believe, feeling he was just saying that to pacify her, giving as her reasons for disbelief that she was too old, too ugly, and too handicapped for anyone to find her sexually desirable. The analyst expressed to the patient his surprise that she herself had, or imagined that he had, values limited to the superficial. He reminded her that their work over many years together had demonstrated to him her inner beauty and deep attractiveness.

For another example, a male patient somewhat younger than his analyst, wondered about his sexual feelings for her. He noted that ordinarily his feelings for her were reciprocated by her feelings for him, and questioned whether this could be true in the erotic realm as well; did she find him sexually attractive? The analyst responded quite simply in the affirmative, because it was true; because it was, as he said, consistent with her general responsiveness to him; and because it was clearly understood between the two of them that their relationship would remain on the level of words. They shared an understanding that erotic feelings are no different than any other feelings, that they can and should be talked about in detail and reflected on without hesitation, when there is no fear that the words would be taken as a seduction toward action.

This case contrasts with another example. Here a male patient told his female analyst early in the treatment that he was only interested in working with a good-looking analyst because he needed her as a subject for his erotic arousal, and that he could not possibly have fantasies or feelings about a less than beautiful woman. The analyst was well able to tolerate and explore these expressions of libidinal interest, but when the patient followed up with questions such as, "What would you do if I were to get up and hug you?" and "Aren't you afraid to be in the same room with a man who could so easily overpower you?" she became more uneasy and found herself less able to maintain her equanimity. She was helped, finally, when the patient asserted, "No matter what you say, I know you are excited by me, too," which assertion put her in touch with the degree to which she felt fear, intimidation, and outrage. The analyst could then respond both authentically and interpretively to the patient's ongoing commentary, fully aware now that these questions all felt to her more like veiled threats than like invitations to exploration or a shared, loving intimacy. She said, "I think I have to make clear to you what I had assumed you already knew, that such actions would not be allowable here; they would interfere with our work." She told him further that to the same degree that he wants to be intimidating to her, she felt uncomfortable with him and did not find him sexually exciting. She then wondered aloud if in his experience he had found women who responded favorably under such circumstances. With some aggression, the patient responded, "Absolutely!" When the patient persisted even more, the analyst informed him that she had decided she could no longer work with him, and she referred him to another analyst, where the work proceeded. In this case for many reasons the analyst had been frightened and put off by the intrusive, aggressive, objectifying tone, more even than by his words, and she realized that although another analyst might have been able to treat the patient as he was, she clearly could not. We want to make clear that it was not the feelings this patient was expressing that led this analyst to stop working with her patient. Rather, it was the threat of impending aggressive sexual action that brought the treatment to a halt.

In yet another case, a male patient entered treatment and almost immediately talked about his sexual attraction to the analyst, commenting on every aspect of her body and being, telling her in great detail exactly what he would like to do with her sexually, how aroused he felt, and how good he could make her feel. He insisted on knowing if the analyst was tempted by this stream of commentary. In fact, the analyst was not, and while respectful of the patient's genuine effort to free associate and to share his feelings, she nevertheless felt that some of what he said was inauthentically erotic, that somehow it did not feel like a sexual interest to her, being mixed with a kind of drivenness. The analyst told the patient that she felt it was more important to understand at that time something about what he felt than to share her own feelings. In part she believed this was true, but in part she did not want to address her own sense that something other than simple erotic attraction was involved. In time they discovered the unconscious re-creation of a past traumatic pattern, in which he had been overstimulated sexually by his alcoholic and disturbed mother. This discovery and its articulation in detail led to diminishment of the driven quality in the patient's sexual expression. The patient was facilitated in his movement out of an old–old relational configuration with himself as a traumatized boy in relation to a sexually traumatizing mother. Ultimately, he was able to enter into a new–new relational configuration, in which he began to feel for the first time what it was like to have his own self needs cared for by an other, rather than being in the care of an other beset by her own problems and whose own needs in the relationship overrode his.

These examples all illustrate instances in which the analyst either responds to the patient's questions about loving and sexual feelings and whether these feelings are returned, or decides not to respond. The decisions are based insofar as possible on what is conceptualized as in the best interests of the patient's development and of the analytic process.

In our view, the relationship between patient and analyst has altered significantly from classical understanding, both in terms of the mutuality and authenticity demanded, and in terms of the range of possibilities that can be safely expressed between them. The relationship we postulate is also altered from an approach that argues for understanding and interpretation from the patient's subjective perspective only, which approach markedly excludes or reduces the analyst's subjective participation as central to the process. Much can be, and often should be, expressed by both patient and analyst directly in words and powerfully in feelings without losing the option for subsequent self-reflection, interpretation, and insight, if these options seem appropriate and helpful to the patient's development. By contrast, in other conceptual models, if something is "gratified," if the analyst responds in a way that addresses that patient's most profound needs or desires, even if only in words, then the opportunity for those longings to be raised to consciousness is conceptualized as forever lost.

To take an extreme example from classical analysis, Mark Kanzer (in Lipton, 1977), in the heyday of ego psychology, chastised Freud for supplying the words "into the anus" for the Rat Man when the Rat Man in their first several sessions together could not bring himself to say them for himself. Kanzer argues that Freud, by speaking his own associations to what he knew the Rat Man could not say and finishing the Rat Man's sentence for him, was symbolically putting his own penis into the Rat Man's anus in the form of those words that Freud had supplied. Freud thereby had gratified the Rat Man's presumed wish for such an anal penetration, and thus, by implication, Freud, with his incautious and spontaneous response, had lost, perhaps forever, the opportunity of analyzing this important unconscious wish of his patient's. With a theory that demands such caution, based on a postulated and ever-incipient risk of permanently spoiling the necessary analysis of crucial drive derivatives, one cannot possibly simply say to the patient as did the analyst in our first example, "I love you, too." The entire analysis would once and for all be rendered useless by virtue of the patient's drive derivatives being gratified, discharged, and hence never to reach secondary process language, so never to be analyzed.

The field has come a long way since organizing technique based on drive theory was in total ascendance. Object relations, self psychology, intersubjectivity, and interpersonal and relational theories, to name but a few, have all made significant contributions to a modification of technique, based on different theoretical systems that regard analysis as a two-person enterprise, with the analyst's participation being viewed not only as inevitable, but as optimal and eminently useful. Yet in these theories, there remains a tendency to sustain a baseline analytic stance in which enactment and provision still pertain. There is a hint that the analyst is doing something unusual, apart from ordinary technique, in response to the patient in such instances. It has been our combined experience in doing supervision and hearing presentations that too often a frank and open sharing of sexual feelings expressed by the patient toward the analyst is met by the analyst's interpreting away from these feelings toward areas that are more acceptable to himself or herself and to the analytic community. In response to the patient's insistent demand to know whether the analyst has sexual feelings toward the patient, for example, the analyst may either explore and perhaps downtune or invalidate the patient's affect; may look beneath the manifest content to alternative, more latent feelings such as hidden hatred, hidden idealization, or longing for nonsexual responsiveness or some other form of sexualized attachment; or, finally, respond with silence, a nonverbal refusal to enter the dialogue, waiting for the patient to go on. Our point here is *not* that any of these responses are inherently wrong—what is helpful and useful depends upon the nature of the interaction, including the dimension of relatedness assumed to be present as well as many other factors that must be attended to. But beyond that, we would contend that the analyst must be able to draw on his or her capacities to share all feelings when they are developmentally appropriate. To be *unable* to do so is limiting to growth, violating an understanding that development encompasses the full range of human relatedness, any part of which must be permissible in analytic exploration and exchange. To repeat, interpretation of either hidden affect or sexualized attachment may well turn out to be the most accurate understanding of the patient's declarations of love; we are only saying that one must be open also to considering the patient's expressions of love at face value.

In any case, we contend that the analyst must always be present, attuned, and mutually interactive, intent on being with the patient in the relational configuration and dimension of intimacy arising from and embedded in the analytic process, and facilitative of the patient's developmental strivings. In our first example, when the patient says, "I love you," she seems to her analyst in that particular instance to be experiencing a new capacity for interpersonal-sharing intimacy with the analyst, and the analyst, by expressing his own feelings, is participating in both the relational configuration and the developmental longing for interpersonal-sharing intimacy. Moreover, as we indicated earlier, this response is not conceptualized in our framework as a "parameter," as in classical theory, nor as an "enactment" nor a "provision," as in the more current relational theories, but rather as just one of many available ways to relate to the patient, any one of which may be seen as best, depending on the relational configuration emergent in the connection, and no one of which has a permanent, privileged standing in furthering the analysis. This is an aspect of analysis unbound, where boundaries are conceptualized as a function of the system.

To make this point that the preferred way of being for the analyst arises from the dimension of intimacy present, and is not dependent on a baseline stance, we can provide another example wherein a patient says to the analyst, "I love you," and the analyst's response is different from our first illustration, emerging from a different affective connection in the relationship. In this latter case, the patient's revelation was offered within the context of a self-protective struggle against an open expression of emotion toward her analyst. The patient, after obviously battling with herself over whether it was safe to reveal what she was feeling, said, "What I didn't want to say to you is that 'I love you.' " The analyst's response matched his patient's reluctant, clouded, and distanced profession of passion. He found himself feeling quite touched by her feelings and by the courage it took to risk an open expression of her emotions. He replied simply, "I'm very moved by what you tell me." Here the analyst was traversing the same affective gradient as his patient, going in the same affective direction, matching the same level of openness balanced by caution. To have said, "I love you, too," would have been too intense, jumping the gradient of expression, markedly uptuning the patient's affect and so running the risk of overstimulation, and missing or disregarding the need for the self-protectiveness inherent in the patient's remark. Instead, the analyst tempered his own response, influenced by the patient's hesitation, maintaining the comfortable, co-created closeness between them, and neither dampening the patient's tender new feelings toward him with a confrontation or interpretation of her cautiousness, nor overwhelming her with emotion that she could not regulate with safety. The analyst could then feel that he had appropriately matched and joined the patient's self state, expressing and sharing his own feelings in response to his patient's feelings. The analyst had in mind an awareness of his patient's progress and of his own satisfaction in that progress, as well as his own personal pleasure in the new space created in their relationship for mutual sharing. Again, as with Kathy K., wherein the analyst's satisfaction was also derived from the analyst's awareness of her patient's new self-reflective abilities, much like a parent who derives satisfaction from the child's growth, so with this patient the analyst felt a pride and pleasure in what his patient could now allow herself to do, and could now allow in the relationship between them.

The analyst was affirmed in his sense that the right tone of interpersonal-sharing intimacy was achieved because the patient was then moved to tell her analyst in more detail of a previous experience with her first analyst wherein mutual expressions of love had led to disastrous sexual enactment. It took the patient 2 years to be able to reveal fully to her current analyst the details of this story, 2 years before she could completely entrust him with her feelings of love without fearing either that his own needs would take priority, or that he would reject her, regarding her as seductive or intemperate in her response. From our point of view, we would say that for the first 2 years, an old self with old other relational configuration had been unconsciously repeated and maintained in the dyad; the current analyst was still organized by the patient as the first analyst had been, as well as, earlier, her husband and, even earlier, her father. This had been a repeated, mainly unconscious relational pattern, then, in which she in the present was as she in the past had been in relation to men who took advantage of, humiliated, and betrayed her for their own self-centered needs. Heretofore, hints of an old self with new other relational configuration had appeared, with the patient struggling to see her analyst differently, as a person concerned with her needs more than his own, but she could only entertain a view of herself as weak and seductive, as undeserving of her analyst's unselfish, altruistic regard. And, then, at this moment in the analysis, we see, based on the safety and security that had been established between them, a new self with new other relational configuration emerging, wherein the patient is able to experience the analyst as a positive new other, an other who would not view her as responsible for what had happened, as others had done in the past. In this context, she herself could become a new self no longer so fearful and also less guilty within the pattern of this positive new experience.

Perhaps it is important at this point to address the question, How deliberative can the analyst's response actually be in moments of such intensity, when the analyst is obviously moved by the patient's expression of feeling? We can only say that much reflection is accomplished preconsciously, seemingly nonreflectively, and understood fully, if at all, only retrospectively. However, in our model, the bidirectionality of interaction posited as existing in the dyadic system imposes an inevitable entrainment wherein the response is always influenced by the other, with more or less self-reflection in the moment. But the point we want to make is that even when self-reflection is absent, bidirectionality is always in place and effects positively the accuracy, specificity, and attunement of the analyst's response to his or her patient.

Bidirectionality, then, renders the analyst's presence and participation an always active phenomenon, its very ongoingness making it an inevitable part of the analytic process. An analyst presented a paper at a conference many years ago describing a slip he had made in telling his young and attractive female patient that her next appointment time was 2 A.M. the following day (Seleznick, 1965). He was responded to by some members of that panel, and by a significant number in the audience, as having ruined the analysis through his woefully unanalyzed countertransference state with his patient, which he unconsciously intruded into the interaction. It was suggested then that the patient must be transferred and the analyst banished to quarantine and reanalysis, certainly a response that would be much tempered today in many analytic circles. As understood from our model, this slip, although still indicating unconscious intent that must be analyzed, only underscores the inevitable embeddedness in the dyad of the analyst's response. And this more dramatic instance of bidirectionality only highlights what goes on all the time in a well-functioning analytic relationship as feelings are mutually experienced and unconsciously expressed.

At this point we will provide another example of love in an interpersonal-sharing dimension of intimacy, illustrating more extensively how unconscious communication on the part of the analyst is understood and conceptualized within our model. A depressed male patient whose parents had been notably unhappy with one another commented to his female analyst that he knew she was subtly but distinctly interested in him, both as a person and, more pertinently, as a sexually desirable man. He told her as well that he felt she was unhappy with her husband, and that he knew he added with his very presence in her life some essential vitality and interest to her existence. As it happened, the patient's perceptions were absolutely correct on all counts, including his assertions about the analyst's sexual interest in him and, at times, even her sexual arousal in his presence. All of this had been disclosed to the patient, not consciously, not deliberately, and not in words, but through a potent, ongoing, affective resonance between them. Moreover, at other times the patient told his analyst that she seemed sad to him and that he felt sorry for her, that he wished to comfort her, and knew that she really desired his comfort, and that she would, despite herself, like a romantic involvement with him, but that both understood that such an affair was out of the question.

On her side, the analyst knew that he knew all of this, and not through deliberate self-disclosure on her part. Moreover, she appreciated the patient for knowing it, felt a poignancy in the intimacy of their relationship, and was able to use all of this to respond in a respectful way that did not deny the patient's reality and yet showed an optimal restraint (M. Shane & Shane, 1996). This analyst could have interpreted her patient's sense of her own unhappiness with her husband as the patient's transference, as, in effect, a displacement from his own parents' obviously troubled marriage, the parents' marriage having been a subject much under discussion in the analysis heretofore, but she chose more authentically to stay with him in the here-and-now, despite her own discomfort at being so exposed without having meant, at least consciously, to reveal herself. This decision was based on her cognizance of the patient's emergent capacity to relate more fully in the interpersonal-sharing dimension of intimacy, and his new ability to resonate accurately with her self state. She proceeded therefore to explore his experience of their relationship, never denying his reality and perceptiveness concerning her own feelings, and in fact validating his sense of his importance to her. This analyst, while appreciative of her patient's needs for a self-transforming connectedness, a need that indeed had been most important throughout most of the treatment, did not mistake the particular instance of interpersonal-sharing intimacy and mutuality for a need on her patient's part for the provision of self-transforming functions. She did not make the mistake, either, despite her own feelings of shame and exposure, of attempting to protect herself or her patient from the effects of the involuntary self-disclosure of her own private longings; doing so would not only have been dishonest and inauthentic, but it most likely would have led to a harmful disruption in the analytic process, disrupting, thereby, the patient's development.

This last clinical vignette illustrates the emerging interpersonal-sharing dimension, wherein the analyst, by unconsciously and nonverbally sharing her own feelings with the patient, demonstrates the powerful effects of bidirectionality. Again, this emergence of a new pattern of intimacy was based in the security of relatedness the patient felt with his analyst, and again, it represented a positive new experience, an experience, therefore, not transference based but based instead on a capacity for novel perceptions of self and other.

THE DIMENSIONS ILLUSTRATED FROM NONANALYTIC LITERATURE

To illustrate that these dimensions of intimacy pertain not just in the clinical situation, but can be found as useful in life and in literature as well, we can use examples from biography and from the short story. We begin with Dierdra Bair's (1990) elegant biography of Simone de Beauvoir.*

The relationship between Jean Paul Sartre and de Beauvoir represents a major focus of this biography. Here is the skeleton of their story. Each had defined the other as the primary and essential relationship for over 50 years, though they had had no sexual contact between them after 8 to 10 years of their knowing one another. Throughout their long relationship, Sartre had confided in de Beauvoir every intimate detail of his own sexual life with a long string of women, seeking her help in facilitating the relationships, in making him feel better about them, or in helping him to end them. These

---

*A different reading of this relationship, along with the case examples of Kathy K. (appearing earlier in this chapter) and the two lawyers (appearing in Chapter 5), is presented in modified form and different conceptualization in *Psychoanalytic Inquiry* (E. Shane & Shane, 1997).

revelations of Sartre's affairs, as de Beauvoir had told her biographer, were always very painful to her, but she continued to listen to her friend, to protect him, and to ensure that he felt no discomfort in confiding in her. Moreover, she kept her own sexual life to herself. She remained quiet about her own life because she knew she would hurt him by telling him about herself and her own lovers. So, we have a situation in which Sartre was completely frank and open about *his* private world, having little or no concern about the effect his confidences would have on his trusted and intimate partner, while de Beauvoir revealed little of herself and was concerned to the utmost about her effect on him. Ethel Person, who had discussed this story in a panel on love and intimacy at the Child Development Center in Los Angeles (Person, 1991), had ended her talk with the question, Is this an intimate relationship? She follows this query with the Zen question, Can one hand clap? We would answer in the affirmative to the question, Is this intimacy?, adding that it is intimacy of a particular type, an intimacy in the self-transforming dimension. As for the Zen question, we see two hands very much in operation, but operating on an unequal participatory basis, each clapping according to its ability and according to its function in the dyad. Sartre uses de Beauvoir as a self-transforming other; he tells her of his private erotic life and, in so doing, uses her to support his shaky self-esteem, to restore his sense of competence vis-à-vis women, to strengthen his self-cohesion and self-consolidation, and whatever else he requires for effective maintenance of his self. The point is, he was not confiding in his intimate friend mindful of her needs or considerate of her feelings but only with an effort to make himself feel better. On the other hand, and in great contrast to her partner, de Beauvoir seems to have been able to consider Sartre's feelings and to regard them as more important to her than her own in this area. She was able to see his separate personhood and agency, keeping in mind the centrality of creating in him a positive sense of comfort and well-being. Apparently there was some pleasure for herself, and perhaps a sense of competence as well, in being able to provide so adeptly for him.

In contrast to this drama, we present O. Henry's (1906/1984) touching and classic story in which two lovers, poor but brimming with an equally developed affection and regard for the other, attempt to solve the problem of giving where there is so little material means to give. Because they have lived lives so closely shared, and have talked so openly with one another, each knows of the other's fondest dreams and each wants more than anything to provide what the other desires. The woman has long, lovely hair that her lover cherishes, and she longs for a decorative comb to adorn it. The comb is expensive, of course, but perfectly suited to her tresses. The man has a gold watch, meaningful to him but which he cannot wear because it lacks a gold chain. He would very much like to have such a chain, but again, the chain is expensive. We all know the bittersweet result. In a poignant gesture, she cuts off her hair, and sells it to purchase the gold chain; he, in a simultaneous gesture, sells his watch in order to buy the comb his lover can no longer use. In this exchange of love and giving, this "Gift of the Magi," the intimate dreams and desires were known and responded to. We cite this as an example of the interpersonal-sharing dimension of intimacy.

To provide a parallel of the Magi story taken from the analytic situation, a patient who was very grateful for changes that had taken place during the course of a long analysis wondered what the analyst would remember of her, as she remembered so much of him. The analyst reminded her that she, a fan of *Alice in Wonderland*, in which half-birthdays are the rule, had told him that St. Patrick's day was the analyst's half-birthday. This gift, he told her, he would remember for the rest of his life, and it would always remind him of her. This was an intimate moment between them, similar in feeling to, but obviously on a different level than, the exchange of gifts in the O. Henry (1906) story. What the pair in O. Henry's story got as the most precious of gifts was the knowledge that each was loved by the other; what the pair in the analytic dyad got was something similar and equally meaningful, but on a level closer to what can be appropriately exchanged in the analytic venue. Again, there was a shared exchange of love, but the general ambience was geared toward and remained focused on the patient's developmental needs even in the context of an interpersonal-sharing intimate exchange.

THE LISTENING POSITION

Finally, we arrive at the listening position that emerges in this developmental systems self psychology approach. We can say most succinctly that the particular way in which we "listen" to the patient, that is, the multiple ways in which the patient is perceived and responded to in the analytic situation, is very much determined by the mutually influencing, bidirectional dimension of intimacy reflected in the dyad, that is, the patient's coming-into-being and coming-into-connection with the analyst. The listening position is also determined, as we have already begun to explore, and as we will describe more fully in the following chapters, by the relational configuration that exists in the moment. First, we want to highlight that we listen to the patient always with the goal, or value, in mind of facilitating the patient's development toward self-consolidation and consolidation of the intimate tie to the other. To this end, we identify components, expectations, actions, patterns, and outcomes that we believe will create the conditions for the emergence of these goals in the treatment process. Second, we want to be clear that we ascribe the status of metaphor to the concept of listening itself—that listening from this developmental systems self psychology perspective invokes all the ways of being with the patient encompassed in our theory, including hearing the patient's subjective experience; interpreting the out-of-awareness meanings the analyst can infer from such subjective reflections; articulating to oneself and perhaps to the patient the intersubjective confluence and affective resonance perceived in the interpersonal connection; reflecting on the nonverbal and physiological concomitants, cues, and procedural aspects of communication in the dyad; potentiating the ongoing self- and mutual-regulatory processes; and, in general, becoming aware of the state of the patient's self, as well as the self-protective strategies invoked by the patient, along with the strategies invoked to preserve the intimate tie to the other. All of these aspects cohere in the analyst's determination of how to listen and to respond optimally, that is, with the goal in mind of establishing the positive new experience for the patient, which will further the consolidation of self and of self with other.

At the core it is essentially as George Eliot has written in *Daniel Deronda* (1874–1876, p. 512): "I begin to think we can only get better having people around us who raise our good feelings."

CHAPTER FOUR

Reconceptualizing Transference

We have indicated that we do not conceptualize the forms of close connection described in our dimensions of intimacy as transference based. Rather we view these connections as aspects of the positive new experience that is the major fulcrum of psychoanalytic change in our model and, we would speculate, the common ground on which all analytic improvement rests, regardless of the analyst's theoretical persuasion.

In this chapter we reconceptualize transference. In all psychoanalytic theories transference encompasses experiences in the present predominantly organized by the past. This contrasts with our concept of positive new experience, which encompasses developmental opportunities new in the patient's life. The understanding of transference as dominated by past relational patterns began with Freud (1912), who declared that what separates psychoanalysts from all other investigators of the human mind is their conviction regarding the etiological significance of early childhood experience to later pathological states. In this view, childhood experience is carried forward, transferred, to the relationship with the analyst. Although the transference concept still remains central in the great majority of psychoanalytic frameworks, it has become extended, expanded, and changed in definition so that, in some ways, its communicative value has been diminished. It has been stretched over time and through a variety of influences coming from the multiple perspectives extant in the field, so that the way in which transference is defined is decisively affected by the frame of reference being invoked. In this chapter we will examine these expanded meanings, separating them out for consideration so that the various usages of the term can be explored and clarified. As will be seen, we make a case for retaining the original, more limited definition of transference—that is, relational patterns dominated by the past— hoping in this way to provide some conceptual clarity for a concept that is vital to psychoanalytic process. Moreover, through this means other aspects buried in the term, which are indispensable in their own right, can be more easily understood and accounted for as to their roles and contributions to the psychoanalytic situation. We have separated out for consideration here three elements often encompassed in current usages of the term "transference." These elements include the following:

1. Transference as a fantasized distortion of past as compared to transference as an accurate (real) reflection of the past.
2. Positive experience as transference experience as compared to positive experience as new experience.
3. Transference as an opportunity for interpretation and insight with ensuing structural change as compared to transference as an opportunity for developmental progression.

As we will clarify, in our model we assume the strategy of conceiving of transference per se rather narrowly. It is only one of three relational configurations that evolves in the analytic situation, all three of which are descriptive of the mutual bidirectional influence of past and present, old and new, within the analytic relationship. Transference is primarily experience based on old patterns, whereas the other two relational configurations we conceptualize include aspects of the positive new experience. We recognize three different relational configurations, rather than conceptualizing transference as the generic term that constitutes the totality of the analytic relationship. The rationale for this latter definition, which expands transference to include *everything* that transpires in the relationship between patient and analyst, is that doing so circumvents the undeniably thorny issue concerning the practical and philosophical difficulties inherent in any attempt to distinguish real from distorted and past from present. Although we appreciate these difficulties, we nevertheless take a different approach. We contend that on a day-to-day basis in the clinical situation itself, these distinctions are always being made by the clinician, whether recognized and acknowledged or not. They are a part of all analytic treatment. As a simple example, interpretations addressing what is presumed to be unconscious ordinarily refer back to a past (if only a recent past) at which time some pattern, content, or configuration was of necessity rendered unconscious. As another example, the basic assumption that childhood experience influences current adult functioning also ordinarily refers back to a past that may influence the present in distorted and confusing ways. Thus, in each of these instances an unstated time dimension is invoked, along with an unstated assumption that past and present can be differentiated.

With these considerations, we limit and confine our own definition of transference. In the relational configuration for which we reserve the term, to be described more fully below, the classical view of transference can be perceived, wherein the past does more than infuse the present, as we agree it inevitably must; it seems to overwhelm it. Transference in our model, then, describes a relational configuration wherein there is a predominance of old patterning over new, that is, of assimilation over accommodation (Piaget & Inhelder, 1969; Slap & Slap-Shelton, 1991). Further, we elect to separate out from transference the other two relational configurations to be described in this chapter, in order to avoid the muddle, to be addressed below, of too much being lumped together under one concept. By taking the route we have chosen, separating out transference from other modes of relating in the analytic situation, we hope to offer a more discrete and descriptive use of the term.

THE CONCEPT OF TRANSFERENCE IN PERSPECTIVE

To review, we are separating out of transference four elements. The first, dimensions of intimacy, was discussed in the previous chapter. The other three to be discussed in this chapter are transference as fantasized distortion of the past versus transference as accurate reflection of the past, positive experience as transference experience versus positive experience as new experience, and transference as an opportunity for interpretation and insight with ensuing structural change versus transference as an opportunity for developmental progression. From our perspective, these four elements are variously conflated within the past-influencing-the-present concept of transference, and therefore require clarification.

The Fantasized/Distorted versus the Accurate/Real

Historical Perspective

We can trace historically the ways in which those elements that act to confuse the original, basic concept of transference have been thought about in the literature. In terms of the real, Freud had taken this aspect of the relationship for granted. He assumed that the analyst could tell what was real in the patient's reactions to him and distinguish it from what was distorted by transference, noting that the patient is "thrown out of the real relationship" by the strength of that transference experience (Freud, 1912, p. 107). As for the patient, from Freud's perspective, for the most part the neurotic individual required the analyst's interpretations to address and rectify reality confusions, a different view than that which holds in today's analysis, wherein reality would most likely be conceptualized as a negotiation between the pair (Gill, 1982). In contrast, it was very clear in Freud's day: The analyst knew what was real and the patient did not, but when the analyst pointed out to the patient what was real, along with explaining how the patient distorted the present stemming from experiences in the past, the patient then knew what was real, as well.

The concept of the real relationship as distinct from and distinguishable from the transference relationship began to slip away when increasing numbers of analysts came to feel that there was no such thing as a conflict-free sphere of the ego, an idea that had been convincingly promoted by Hartmann (1950) and Rapaport (1960a, 1960b), leaders of the ego psychology that had held sway in this country until the 1970s. In contrast, many analysts had come to believe that all aspects of the relationship were suffused with unconscious conflict. With no nonconflictual relationship, then, there could be no clearly real relationship that could be reliably separated out from transference infusion (Brenner, 1982; Stein, 1981). The strategy then became, as noted above, to call *all* aspects of the relationship between patient and analyst "transference," thereby avoiding the reality question in the relationship altogether. This strategy is observable in much contemporary theory, including Kleinian, object relational, classical, self psychological, interpersonal relational, and intersubjectivity, so that the issue of real versus distorted in the analytic relationship becomes a nonissue, not requiring solution: The whole relationship is suffused with transference. The holdouts who still distinguish transference from nontransference in the analytic situation include Modell (1988), Kernberg (1988), those who retain the concept of the therapeutic alliance (e.g., Schlessinger & Robbins, 1983) , many child analysts (e.g., A. Freud, 1966), and many other classical analysts. For this group, the problem of the real, which may likely be negotiated in the dyad or arbitrarily decided by the analyst (à la Freud), also does not require solution.

From our perspective, one reason for narrowing our definition of transference and thus, apparently, moving against the contemporary trend, is that reality has a very important place in our theory, and not just as it pertains to the analytic relationship. It becomes essential from our perspective to be able to address all aspects of the question concerning what is real: Where is the place for distortion? Where is the place for the question, Did it really happen? What is the relation between "the real" and "the sense of the real"? These are issues that are submerged, we think, when the view of transference is expanded to include all experience, conflating such important distinctions.

Developmental Systems Self Psychology Perspective

Although philosophers have struggled for centuries to grasp and master the concept of the real, one current approximation that we can adopt for the purposes of our framework has been offered by Marcia Cavell (1993) and Donald Davidson (1986). Each posits that reality can be accepted as a cultural given in the individual's development, understood broadly as an unconscious consensus agreed upon in the culture and reflected in the individual as a sense of what is real. In addition, we are helped by the scientific perspective on reality, which postulates that a reality exists apart from what we can know about reality through any theories or experiments that we might construct. That is, there is an underlying assumption in science of a model-free reality, or to use Hawking's (1988) term, a "model-independent reality" (pp. 44–45), that is, a reality existing apart from the theoretical postulates that are designed to explain it. In this sense, science can only approximate what is real, for reality can only be known through theoretical construction or conjecture.

This scientific assumption of a model-independent reality has clinical relevance and importance if we use it as an agreed-upon construct: Individuals can only know about their world through their own sense impressions, but nevertheless there is a world out there that exists independent of these impressions but is reflected, more or less, in them. Through this construct, the pervasive confusion that exists between what is real for the patient subjectively, and what really happened to that patient "objectively," can be approached. The importance of this distinction from our perspective lies in the fact that reconstructions, co-constructions, and re-creations, as discoverable through the hermeneutics of the clinical situation based on the patient's and the analyst's subjective and intersubjective experiences and attributions of meaning, can derive important substance, direction, limitation, and constraint through the analyst's knowledge and clinical use of knowledge from many areas outside of the patient–analyst dyad. These areas include brain formation and function, normal emotional development, and cognitive development, all of which are also only approximations of a model-independent reality. Here we can see the inevitable interconnection between sense of reality, that is, what feels real for the individual, and the construct of a model-independent reality, that is, reality independent of the individual's unique perspective, what is "out there" and consensually validated, not just by patient and analyst, but also by findings of a wider scientific community. For some, such a connection may seem unimportant, because there are no absolute answers to the questions, is it real? Did it really happen?, and therefore no way to go beyond what is, after all, only subjective reality. For us, on the other hand, it is important to acknowledge the interconnection between the real and the sense of the real, while at the same time preserving their difference, recognizing that each is a separate entity and a separate way of conceptualizing one's experience of the real. Indeed, the real and the sense of the real appear to us as conceptually distinguishable and yet as interconnected in the system, as is the self and the other in the selfother system, or as two subjectivities in an intersubjective system. That is, the self and the other, like the two subjectivities in the intersubjective field, "exist" importantly both as individual entities and as interconnecting entities, both as essentially separate and distinct in their own right and as essentially intertwined within the system. So it is, we believe, with the "real" and the sense of the real.

A clinical example illustrates this important connection between the real (as model-independent reality) and the sense of the real (as idiosyncratic, subjective experience). The knowledge concerning the connection between dissociative flashback experience and trauma, as evidenced in the work of researchers such as van der Kolk, McFarlane, and Weisaeth (1996) and Pynoos and Eth (1985), contributes an understanding of the probable connection between these particular manifestations appearing in the present in the clinical situation and the likelihood of real trauma having occurred at some point earlier in the patient's life. Such flashback experience typically takes the form of procedurally mediated bodily phenomena accompanied by expressions of inexplicable, nameless, inchoate fear or dread. These procedural memories are unavailable in declarative, symbolic, verbalizable, subjective experience, either to the patient's conscious mentation or to the patient's dynamically unconscious mentation. Yet they are powerful manifestations that must be understood.

Such clinically derived evidence, matched by findings from the empirical literature, raises the likelihood of real life trauma having occurred in the patient's past as opposed to having the status of fantasized creations or distortions on the part of the patient. Such matching of clinical observation and empirical data addresses the questions, Is it real? Did it really happen? How do we come to any workable conclusion about this dilemma? It is important to emphasize that such manifestations as flashbacks and bodily expressions of fear, which can be observed clinically and are matched by empirical data, cannot be taken as proof of what happened, but rather serve as clues for the direction of future analytic exploration, always constrained, restrained, and redirected in the clinical situation by what emerges subsequently in the analysis.

The above example also may serve to illustrate what is meant when it is posited that reality for the individual is both idiographic and nomothetic. The particular form the dissociative phenomena may take is idiographic, unique to the individual; however, the phenomenon of dissociation itself is an inherent capacity of the self under threatening circumstances, and so may be postulated as nomothetic, lawful and generalizable to the human condition.

We draw on the work of several researchers from diverse fields for hypotheses concerning the sense of the real. We seek to conceptualize how a sense of the real develops and how this sense becomes connected to emerging capacities of the self. We begin with the writings of Gerald Edelman. As noted in Chapter 1, Edelman (1992) distinguishes two kinds of consciousness: primary consciousness and higher-order consciousness. Primary consciousness is the first type of consciousness achieved evolutionarily and by the human infant in development, and, incidentally, it occurs in other primates as well. It is the state of being mentally aware of things in the world, of having mental images in the present. Thus primary consciousness is tied to real time and limited to the chunk of time called the present. Edelman likens the experience of primary consciousness to a flashlight beam that shines in the dark: Only that which is captured and illuminated by the beam is perceived and organized as reality; all else remains in darkness. The illuminated experience constitutes what Edelman calls the "remembered present," by which he means that the perception is remembered and connected with previous experience only in the moment. All experience for the individual who is exclusively dependent on primary consciousness requires for the recall of past experience retrieval cues in the immediate surround. For the clinician, the concept of primary consciousness may provide a model for encoding the heightened moment of experience in which self-reflection does not play a part, for example, the flashback experience itself. This form of consciousness may therefore provide a basis for theorizing about experience that can be recaptured by the individual only in the presence of retrieval cues for revivification of that heightened moment of experience from the past.

How, asks Edelman (1992), is the individual able to overcome this tyranny of the remembered present? This question led Edelman to a consideration of his second kind of consciousness, higher-order consciousness. This latter form of consciousness is, in short, a consciousness of being conscious, a capacity to self reflect. The development of higher-order consciousness is based on the acquisition of language and other means of symbolic, social communication. These acquisitions permit a new ability to distinguish between ongoing events occurring in real time, that is, the remembered present of primary consciousness, from inner life experienced self-reflectively. This allows individuals to present back to themselves their own inner worlds now available to them symbolically. There is thus a reorganization of past as well as present experience, distinguishable from immediate perception. An inner life with higher-order consciousness capable of modeling a past, present, and future; a reflective capacity; and a comprehensible world are all rendered possible.

It is here that the nature of lived experience plays such a formative and formidable role, bringing in the importance of the attachment bond, the importance of the type of attachment achieved and available to the individual. With secure attachment, self-reflective capacities are enhanced (Fonagy, Steele, Steele, Moran, & Higgitt, 1991) and past and present, real and unreal, become more easily distinguished. With insecure attachment, self-reflection is compromised, and hence, too, the capacities for distinguishing past from present and real from distorted in the autobiographical narrative (Main & Goldwyn, 1985). In the clinical situation, the individual with a secure attachment is able to take in an interpretation of these distinctions, and to reflect on it. When the analyst says, "You seem to be afraid that I will abandon you as others in your life have done," the patient can hear and profit from an underlying knowledge that, at least in part, the analyst is not like the abandoning others from the past. The analyst and patient can then explore in what ways the analyst is and is not an abandoning other in the patient's life. In contrast, the person who is locked in a transference configuration, experiencing the past as overwhelming and overriding the present, is neither likely to be accessible to interpretations of such distinctions, nor likely to be able to participate in an exploration of such feelings. This familiar clinical dilemma is in part what has led us to look beyond interpretation for help when interpretation fails. Hence, whereas higher-order consciousness and concomitant self-reflection are ordinarily available as functional capacities, in the highly charged emotional relationship with the analyst, where old patterns may emerge in the present context, higher-order consciousness and self-reflective awareness are compromised.

Moreover, the higher-order consciousness existing in the individual is idiosyncratic, so that the individual's subjective sense of reality is also idiosyncratic. Yet the presence of this consciousness does allow the individual the potential for approaching a consensually validated reality through interconnections with others; the individual sense of reality can thus be shared with, and moreover is dependent on, an embeddedness in the environment. In summary, a full development of the individual, both phylogenetically and ontogenetically, entails the maturation of a capacity to self-reflect, to know the world subjectively, to appreciate the subjectivity of the other as compared with one's own, and, finally, to achieve a sense of reality that has consensual consistency with and is therefore constrained by the surround. Yet these capacities, although usually present to some degree, can be compromised by constitutional and experiential difficulties.

This higher-order consciousness, allowing for a sense within the self of past, present, and future, is connected to continuity of the self, an important component of self-integration and self-consolidation. The self that has been subjected to trauma, as in the example of the patient above who dissociates, is lacking just such a sense of continuity. The flashback, although really happening within the individual and revivified in the present, is without the time perspective provided by higher-order consciousness and self-reflective awareness, thus disturbing a sense of self-continuity. The self-protective (defensive) strategy of dissociation, so necessary at the time of the original trauma, prevents the symbolic encoding of the event, interfering with the ordinary functioning of higher-order consciousness, and in effect keeping this event encoded only in primary consciousness. The result is a self lacking both in continuity and in a stable sense of the real.

Transference in our model reflects exactly this condition. We postulate transference as a relational configuration in which the patient's self is not consolidated, past and present cannot be distinguished, and real and distorted are confused. A secure attachment, which permits a coherent life narrative, enhanced self-reflection, and capacity for firm reality testing, is unavailable to the patient in this transferential relational configuration. The other two configurations we have identified in our model describe the developmental trajectory that moves the patient from the condition of being locked in the past, without effective time perspective, self-continuity, or self-reflective capacity, along to conditions in which such time perspectives and such self-reflective capacities are facilitated in the relationship with the analyst.

Edelman's (1992) neurophysiological model of the real, which informs our view of transference, is consistent also with Stern's (1985) developmental model of the real. Stern writes that the infant is at first reality bound, linked to real experience, and is an accurate recorder of that real experience, to the limits of his or her cognitive capacity, remaining limited to that reality perception until the infant acquires the ability to symbolize. The emergence of the symbolic capacity allows the developing individual to create an inner world that transcends reality, though still deriving from it, freeing him or her from a reality-bound state. Now the developing child can amend reality for his or her own purposes, creating thereby a world more tolerable to the self. And with the symbolic capacity, the child can be expressive in what we identify as two different modes, which become elaborated over the lifespan and become relevant clinically. The first is the realm of *self-protection*, and the second is the realm of *creative self-elaboration*. These modes, although different, do intertwine in mutual influence.

In terms of the mode of self-protection, the individual can now use the new capacities for symbolic function to cope with the reality of the selfsurround, or, in more familiar psychoanalytic parlance, to distort that reality for deliberate, defensive purposes. It is important from our perspective to make a distinction between the two kinds of self-protective strategies now available: those earlier strategies that arise procedurally, which are not mediated symbolically, and those later-evolved strategies that depend on the new symbolic capacity.

Once available in development, both strategies are used throughout life.

In the procedural category we can name three prototypes of self-protection: first, those protections found in the very young infant, in the form of aversive withdrawal; second, those protections arising in the last quarter of the first year of life, taking the form of the attachment patterns first recognized through the Ainsworth (1982) Strange Situation; and, third, those protections occurring at any age in response to trauma, resulting in the formation within the self of multiple, not fully integrated, nonverbal self states. In the symbolically mediated category are self-protective strategies such as the familiar defenses of disavowal, repression, reaction formation, and the like. In our framework, we define as self-protective any strategy, either procedurally or symbolically mediated, generated by the self in response to traumatic circumstances. All of these strategies represent means to deal with real experiences that are too painful to integrate, and that have interfered with self-consolidation.

The second mode we identify, the mode of creative self-elaboration, is made available by the attainment of symbolic capacity. The individual with symbolic capacity is enabled not only to remember and to reflect, as discussed above, but also to imagine what is not real and to elaborate an inner world unique to and expressive of the self. In this mode, play and imaginative invention evidence the creativity of the individual, along with the use of such self-protective strategies as denial in fantasy and intellectualization, which are examples of the potential for intertwining creative self-elaboration with self-protection.

Here Edelman's (1992) concept of "bootstrapping" is relevant. In common usage, bootstrapping is a metaphor that refers to pulling oneself up by one's own bootstraps, by which is meant the nearly impossible capacity to help oneself without the aid of others and to rely entirely on one's own efforts and resources. In Edelman's concept, bootstrapping connotes a kind of self-elaboration not based on perception of the world in the moment, but based instead on the individual's unique and original conceptual recategorization of that world taking place entirely within the self. Edelman uses the concept of bootstrapping to help explain the diversity in human beings, for example, to explain how siblings raised in the same family by the same caregivers can be so different from one another. This concept of bootstrapping seems relevant clinically because it frees us from postulating development of self, including both self-protective and creative self-elaborative strategies, as being exclusively modeled on either gene makeup or on the relational tie to the other. In this way, the development of the self is freed from inevitable bondage either to inborn characteristics or to influences of individuals in the surround. It leaves room for totally new, novel, unique characteristics arising as if out of nowhere from within the individual, setting him or her totally apart from others in the family. The concept of bootstrapping requires a nonlinear dynamic systems understanding. It explains how the individual is both independent and interdependent in functioning, and both isolated and interconnected in creativity and in self-protection. A systems perspective, then, permits a contextualized comprehension of the individual both as a subjective entity and as an intersubjective unity, in both one-person and two-person perspectives.

A short clinical example concerns a creative individual who in childhood had attempted to lock himself in his room to avoid his excruciatingly intrusive mother. However, she had insisted that his makeshift locks be removed for her own free entry, and she barged into his room indiscriminately. The boy thus had no other recourse for self-protection than to retreat into his own head. Here, hunkered down as if in a bunker, he created his own unique world. It was years later that he was able to share this world with the public as a novelist, to great acclaim. He found himself so alienated from his family of origin that he suffered a kind of survival guilt, which subsequently brought him into analysis. This self-contained, autotelic universe the boy and then the man had created was an instance of bootstrapping. From whence he derived his characters and his fictional world remained a mystery, untraceable by him and unconnectable to those who raised him. On their part, his family saw him then and see him still as an oddity, totally inexplicable, often wondering aloud to others, in his presence, where on earth this guy, this son and brother, had come from.

To summarize our effort to reconceptualize transference regarding the concept of the real, what is experienced as real both is a property of the organizing perspective of the self (e.g., higher-order consciousness) and is inextricably emergent in interconnection with the surround (e.g., the self-reflective capacity that arises from a secure base). Important to this conception of the real is the contribution of a culturally organized, consensually validated conception of reality. Also contributing are the developing capacities in the individual for creative self-elaboration and for self-protection, capacities that constitute important attributes of a consolidated self but that can become the bases for what appear as distortions in the creation of the life narrative. In the clinical situation, as happened earlier in the family of origin, the analytic dyad creates together a consensually validated sense of what is real, both in the past and in the current situation. Here, too, creative self-elaborative and self-protective strategies contribute, constituting in the clinical situation, as well as in development, a means for self-consolidation. This, from our perspective, is as close as one can get to our ongoing effort to approximate the real, what really happened in the patient's life, and what really happens between patient and analyst, both in the past and in the present.

We will close this discussion with an exchange that took place between Kohut and Anna Freud, which we believe exemplifies the struggle inherent in any attempt to answer the question, Did it really happen, or is it a product of the patient's distortion?

In a letter dated 1967 (in Cocks, 1994), written to Heinz Kohut in response to his sending her a manuscript of his work, Anna Freud admonishes Kohut for, from her perspective, being too focused on past real trauma in patients with narcissistic (self) disturbances, as opposed to recognizing the intrapsychic aspects contributing to the patients' illnesses. We quote this letter at length because Anna Freud addresses Kohut as a friend; as a fellow liberal, theoretically speaking; and as an avowed fellow "environmentalist" in terms of her conviction concerning the influences of the actual environment on child pathology. The letter itself follows by 1 year her definitive book on child analysis (1966) where she had in fact called herself an environmentalist.

> Loss of object in early times, traumatic disappointment in the maternal or parental object: I have to add here that recently I acquired a mistrust of the concepts which are in such wide use now. The terms seem to imply that there were real events in the external world and I think only too often that this is not true. That what exerts an influence are purely internal fluctuations of cathexis. There are, of course, no undisturbed relationships, especially not in childhood where the demands on the object are so unrealistic.
>
> I am thinking here of two of my own patients, both homosexual before their analysis, both narcissistic personalities, one of them besides an addict, the other an obsessional neurosis. Both of them had devoted mothers who never wavered in their attention to them. Both had siblings, and were themselves the youngest, which means that the presence of the sibling was a given, an immutable fact from the begin-

ning, not a traumatic event. In spite of this, they acted as if they had been deserted at some time by the mother, and the addiction quite obviously had to make up for this. What the analysis showed was an inordinate jealousy of the siblings, which turned every attention paid to them by the mother into a traumatic experience. Would you call this a disappointment or loss of the object? In reality it is an inordinate demand with disastrous consequences. Is it a special oversensitiveness and shakiness of object relationship, i.e., a failure of frustration tolerance in this respect? Whatever it is, I believe it should not be confused with a real life experience, such as death, separation, neglect, etc. Is it perhaps a narcissistic quality in the object relationship which turns every slight into a deadly insult?

These are some of my thoughts that accompanied the reading [of Kohut's manuscript copy of what was to be published as *The Analysis of the Self*]. They are not worth very much, but you will take them for what they are: signs of interest in what you are producing. (in Cocks, 1994, p. 184)

In our model, we adopt the developmental and self psychological perspective that if the patient reports an experience from the past as having been traumatic, we are prone to accept that judgment, whether the traumatic nature of the event in question stems directly in response to the event in itself, or from some fantasized elaboration of that event. This clinical assumption applies not just to single, isolated experiences, but to cumulative experiences, as well. Our bias, unlike that of Anna Freud, is that if a patient describes an unavailable mother, there is likely to be some very basic, significant truth in that description, however much the described interactions may have been elaborated through self-protective strategies. Bowlby (1973), writing around the time Anna Freud had written to Kohut (in Cocks, 1994), comments eloquently on this matter: "The varied expectations of the accessibility and responsiveness of attachment figures that different individuals develop during the years of imma-turity are tolerably accurate reflections of the experiences those individuals have actually had" (in Sroufe, 1996, p. 172). In terms of the cases Anna Freud writes about to Kohut, we would say, following Bowlby, that those mothers were the subjects of "tolerably accurate reflections" as made by their children, Anna Freud's patients, and that, in the terms of our model, the patients experienced the trauma that generated the fragility of self from which they suffer, and the entrenched self-protective strategies that were the object of Anna Freud's psychoanalysis.

Positive Experience as Transference Experience versus Positive Experience as New Experience

Historical Perspective

The second element we wish to consider in this process of reconceptualizing transference is the concept of the positive experience as transference, that is, as stemming from past relationships, in contrast to the concept of positive experience as new experience, which is not based on past relationships. Freud (1912) conceptualized the *unobjectionable positive transference* as a means to explain the patient's cooperation with the analyst in the psychoanalytic process. In Freud's terms, the unobjectionable positive transference is defined as the patient's current experience of the analyst based on that patient's early trust and reliance on caregivers in childhood, which is then transferred to the analyst and which Freud advised should be allowed to continue uninterpreted in the present analytic situation. It is this unobjectionable positive transference carrying with it old (nontraumatic) experience that allows a new experience to be constructed in the analysis, a new experience with the caregiving, loved analyst who provides a particular ambience in which new insight and working through can evolve, with new structure resulting. In Freud's model, positive experience in the present analytic situation derives from and builds on similar experiences in the past; that is, there is a template for positive experience available within the patient based on early, good relational patterns with caregivers and/or on already mastered unconscious intrapsychic conflicts. In more contemporary models too, such positive experiences are conceptualized as transference. For example, Kohut (1977) conceptualized the selfobject experience so central to analysis in his model as transference based, a renewed opportunity, largely positive, for the patient to experience with the analyst those functions vital to self-development that were incompletely provided in childhood. Modell (1988) constructed the dependent-containing experience, also central to analysis in his model, as transference based, built on experiences pertaining to infancy and childhood in which the caregiving other could be depended on to contain powerful affects.

Finally, an appreciation for the complexity of past and present mutually influencing each other has led many contemporary analysts to put aside any consideration of a distinction between past and present, old and new, as a defining factor in their consideration of what constitutes either transference or positive experience in the analytic situation. At the same time, they recognize, implicitly or explicitly, the importance of the influence of the patient's past on his or her current life. For us, however, as will be elaborated below and throughout this book, a distinction between past and present, old and new, is crucial. For us, the positive new experience is of central importance in understanding therapeutic action in psychoanalysis, though the distinction between old and new can only be couched in relative terms, and then only as it emerges out of the patient–analyst system. In our view, whether one considers therapeutic action in psychoanalysis to derive solely from past templates of previous experience, or whether one leaves conceptual room for new, never-before-had positive experience, not based on prior relational patterns, will greatly affect one's clinical approach. The unique personhood of the analyst becomes more significant. The analyst, in addition to being a vehicle for evoking past relational patterns, becomes a new person in the patient's life, with the freedom to provide a fuller range of human interaction. We will anticipate the introduction of our own perspective in the following section by providing two short clinical examples of the analyst functioning deliberately as a new person in the patient's life.

An analyst working with a very frightened patient, who suffered from self states that reflected unintegrated core body experience, was convinced that this patient would greatly benefit from some form of ongoing, nonthreatening touch to facilitate a sense of bodily cohesion and a reduction of a feeling of being an alien creature. The analyst had contemplated offering to hold the patient's hand, but, knowing that such a gesture would be much too threatening, that the patient was too fearful of human touch, explored with the patient the idea of the analyst's bringing in her own pet dog to share. This unusual gesture turned out to be helpful to the patient, providing a new experience of being able to relate, and to relate physically, to an embodied being, with the analyst hoping that this capacity would translate to further development.

A second example concerns a patient in the throes of a divorce, who was experiencing spasms of anxiety, sleeplessness, and returns to old states of traumatized helplessness, symptoms that had abated for the past several years. The analyst, feeling sufficient exploration had already taken place in regard to transference meanings and to the patient's current self state, and feeling as well that the picture of the deteriorated condition of the marriage was sufficiently clear, did not hesitate to introduce his own point of view, and his own sense of trust in the patient's capacities and in the work that had already taken place in the analysis. He said to the patient that he believed that the patient's current symptoms were akin to the violent vibrations that accompany movement through the sound barrier for the first time. The analyst told her further that the pilot in this situation needed the confidence to know that despite intense anxiety in the moment, the moment would be lived through, with smooth sailing ensuing once the sound barrier had been broken. This analyst could take this risk because he knew the patient, had a conviction about the process, and understood that the patient required something new from him that would facilitate this important developmental move in her life.

Developmental Systems Self Psychology Perspective

In our framework, as we indicated above, only one of the three relational configurations that we conceptualize as emerging in the selfother dynamic system encompasses the old or the past as the predominant influence on the patient, with the other, the analyst, assimilated into that pattern of old, past experience. We refer to this configuration as transference. Further, we limit the inclusion of the old or past in the relational configuration we refer to as transference to old or past *trauma*, separating out from our definition of transference old or past experiences that were more positive or more neutral in nature, not requiring the adoption of self-protective measures in order to permit the individual to cope with the situation at hand. We contend that these predominantly positive patterns from the past can be integrated into the individual's more general, ongoing self-development, remaining available for future, flexible accommodation and assimilation. In the case of positive patterns, a dialectic is maintained between assimilation of new experience into familiar existent memory of past experience, posed against accommodation of that memory to reflect new, present experience, achieving thereby an equilibrium, a balance, between assimilation and accommodation, past and present in the patient's experience. Trauma, on the other hand, is most often sequestered, not allowing for such flexible accommodation and assimilation. Where there is trauma, higher-order consciousness is compromised, integration of new experience is limited, and self-reflective capacity is much reduced or is absent in relation to these traumatic experiences, so that the present remains assimilated into, and confused with, past sequestered patterns. In effect, then, for a person in a traumatic state, the present does not exist. As a simple but potent example, the patient who experiences periodic, driven bingeing cannot, while in that driven state, recall or draw from the memory of other states or other needs and intentions, nor reflect on the present or future. That patient in that moment of bingeing is living only in the past and in accordance with past imperatives.

Hence, in our model, when a patient experiences the analyst in a manner that would have been described by Freud as a positive unobjectionable transference, or that would be described in self psychological theory in selfobject transference terms or by Modell (1988) in dependent-containing transference terms, we, in contrast, would not categorize such experiences in the patient–analyst system as transference at all. We mean by this that this positive experience on which this aspect of the relationship with the analyst is based does not call for self-protective strategies, is not sequestered, and does not lock either self or other into any particular figure from the past.

For example, when exploring the experience of the patient's positive feelings for the analyst, a connection might be made to a kindly grandfather in the patient's past, and to the patient's self as the loved and protected grandchild, but in our model such a connection is not considered transference: The capacity to feel loved and protected by the other has been integrated into the patient's way of being with an other and remains a pattern that can be repeated in many relationships. Moreover, in this example there would be no necessity for the patient to restrict his view of himself or the analyst to that particular kindly, grandfather–grandchild image; the patient, not being in a transference-based, old self with old other relational configuration, is not blinded to those qualities of self and other in the present that are different from the grandfather–grandchild interactive pattern. Again, these features of flexibility make the experience of the kindly grandfather pattern not transference, but rather a feature of the patient's nontraumatic, healthy self.

We want to make clear, however, that we would not consider these positive, non-transference-based experiences with the analyst built upon healthy aspects of the patient's self as sufficient to constitute meliorative therapeutic action. We contend that drawing on a patient's positive experiences in the past is not sufficient to move the patient along the trajectory of developmental progression toward self-consolidation. The provision of positive *new* experiences is likely to be necessary, based on what the patient cannot yet know and cannot yet do if left only to his or her own past experience and already developed healthy capacities. The goal in our model, as we indicated earlier, is to encourage freedom and creativity in the patient–analyst pair to seek out ways to enhance development within the analytic situation.

To continue along this same line, we do not mean to say that all the patient's positively toned experiences of the analyst are to be considered nontransferential and nontraumatic in their origins. Were the patient unable to see the analyst in any other terms but the most benign, one might suspect that a self-protective strategy was in place, necessitated by a response to past trauma, the analyst being confined by the patient to a positive view in order to defend against fearful and/or forbidden anger, for example. In our model, such a purely positively toned pattern would be conceptualized as transference, a pattern experienced in the analytic relationship, which had been sequestered defensively in the past to protect the self against danger.

In our model, then, we reserve the term *transference* for trauma-togenic patterns stemming from the patient's past and reexperienced in the treatment. These experiences in our model are ultimately interpreted and/or lived through in the analytic relationship. As to the question addressed above of what to do with positive feelings, in our model we distinguish two possible pathways, depending on the circumstances that pertain. Following one pathway, the positive relationship to the analyst is put into words and interpreted as possibly hiding other feelings. The patient's positive feelings are explored by the analyst for any defensive disguises they might provide. Along this pathway all such feelings are examined analytically, helping the patient to get in touch with any ambivalence or alternative self states that may be currently kept from awareness. Following a second pathway, the analyst posits that the patient's positive feelings should be fostered and allowed to evolve without interruption. Here the analyst is concerned to avoid a potential disruption in a positively evolving developmental sequence and is motivated to allow such feelings to be elaborated.

In our systems model, the determination of which pathway to follow depends on specific circumstances in the current analytic relationship. Such circumstances include the dimension of intimacy present in the foreground, as was described in the previous chapter, as well as the configuration emerging in the relationship, and the currently perceived trajectory of developmental progression, which latter topics are only referred to in this chapter, but will be described more fully in the next. In the example that follows, we focus on an instance wherein positive affect is conceptualized as transference because it is perceived to be used self-protectively by the patient, embedded in a traumatic pattern of relatedness stemming from the past. Hence, in this instance the expression of positive affect is explored and interpreted.

A patient from time to time reported to his analyst that he was feeling much better as a result of the work the pair had been doing, but the analyst could not help but note on some occasions a shameful, guilty expression playing across the patient's face and hints of the patient's unacknowledged anxiety. It took some time for the analyst to identify a pattern assuming shape in the analysis. The pattern consisted of the patient's words expressing positive feelings, in the form of appreciation for the analysis and a sense of closeness to the analyst, accompanied by a particular expression on the patient's face, the combination having the effect of warning the analyst that all might not be as the patient had said, or that certain experiences were being left unsaid. The analyst was thus alerted to an increase in apprehension on the patient's part, evidenced by requests for affirmation from the analyst, a requirement for reassurance that the analyst, too, felt that things were going well. On his part, the analyst would note feeling uncharacteristically irritated with these demands for reassurance, and a sense that to respond as the patient wished would have the effect of placing him in a false position. The entire pattern, repeated several times, conveyed ultimately to the analyst a conviction that he might need to put into words for the patient his sense that things were not as they seemed. What was uncovered in the dialogue that followed and was then interpreted was that the patient, whenever he felt a loss of connection to the analyst, would return to an old habit of drinking and would feel momentary shame and guilt in response, resulting in a greater loss of connection, both to himself and to the analyst. The disavowed loss of connection was based on an unconscious anticipation of the analyst's judgment and criticism, so that the patient would be moved to seek reassurance without any awareness of why he was doing so. The patient's request for affirmation from the analyst would then be met by a palpably distant analyst instead of the warm, reassuring analyst the patient wished for. By fully exploring this sequence, it was discovered that the patient's outward show of positive feelings was embedded in an old relational configuration with his father wherein the requirement to keep the tie to the other (now the analyst) entailed the presentation of a perfect facade: Thus, the patient had to conform and to comply, to present a false front, as would surely be required by the traumatogenic parent/analyst based on the patient's experience of his father in the past.

The point we are making is that it is not the quality of the presenting affect per se that determines whether what is being experienced with the analyst represents a positive experience (nontransferential in our model) stemming from earlier in the patient's life versus a negative, traumatic experience (transference in our model) stemming from an earlier period. Rather, it is the extent to which that positive affect apparent in the analytic situation is reflective of a consolidated self and embedded in a secure, intimate tie to an other, or whether it is reflective of a self-protective strategy designed to ward off unacceptable affect states and to prevent a repetition of the original trauma. This important distinction between a positive affect that is transference based, and a positive affect that is a part of a healthy consolidated self, can often only be known through emergent experience in the analysis, as we have just illustrated.

We have no wish to convey that all positive affect covers over a hidden affect, hidden because it is objectionable in Freud's terms. Nor, on the other hand, do we wish to convey, because there is positive affect apparently reflective of a consolidated self and a consolidated intimate tie, that no further inquiry need be made. In contrast, in our model it is important for analyst and patient to recognize together and to explore at times even these apparently felicitous states. On the other hand, if the analyst does not have within his or her theory conceptual space for acknowledging a healthy configuration when it does exist, that configuration can be misunderstood and misinterpreted as a self-protective strategy, as Kohut (1971) has exemplified many times. For example, Kohut describes how an analyst disrupts a patient's healthy idealizing experience when he assumes as inevitable the existence of hidden aggression, and then interprets that aggression. If the patient then erupts in anger, feeling misunderstood, the analyst may take it as confirmation of his theoretical assumption, not being aware that what has just occurred is an instance of the analyst's provoking in the patient the very aggression he had so confidently postulated, an aggression in Kohut's theory that was actually in reaction to the patient's experience of feeling poorly understood.

As a variant of this same kind of clinical misjudgment delineated by Kohut (1971), based on the theoretical assumption that all of the patient's attitudes toward the analyst are obligatorily ambivalent, we can cite a situation frequently encountered in analysis: A patient, while relating to the analyst in a comfortable, intimate mode, tells the analyst about feelings of disappointment and anger with an important person in the patient's life. It is commonplace for analysts to think in terms of the patient's displacement away from the relationship with the analyst in such situations; that is, when the patient speaks of others in the analytic hour, the reference to the other serves as a disguise for the patient's unconscious feelings of a similar nature toward the analyst. The risk in automatically assuming and interpreting such displacement is that of putting oneself in the position Kohut describes, potentiating a disruption of a secure attachment. However, were one automatically to accept and never interpret such potential displacement, then one would risk making the patient feel misunderstood in another direction.

How does the analyst make the decision of which direction to follow? It is complex, of course, but it helps to leave open the possibility of both alternatives, based on a sense that good feelings toward the analyst are not necessarily transference based, nor all feelings expressed toward an other always necessarily ambivalent. This openness in the analyst, together with his or her clinical self-trust and knowledge of the patterns that are familiar in this particular dyad, gives the analyst a better likelihood of understanding correctly in the moment what the patient means in depth. In our developmental systems self psychology approach, we presume that the meanings of the patient's comments will emerge of a piece with a sense of mutual conviction, with the possibility always present that both patient and analyst can be proven wrong in the future. Again, assurance lies in trust in one's mutual conclusions, another marker of secure attachment in the pair existing for at least that chunk of time. Assurance also lies in a capacity to be proven wrong if the circumstances dictate. Where secure attachment pertains, both patient and analyst can expect a curiosity, a confidence, a willingness to explore, and an expectation that one's affects, painful or not, will be welcomed and responded to. These are highly important moments in the analysis from our perspective, not to be dismissed as merely unobjectionable or nonconflictual, but rather to be drawn on when the analysis, as it most likely will, evokes another, less hopeful, more painful facet stemming from the patient's past or current experience. In this vein, periods of mutual secure attachment can serve as an antidote to the patient's crushing hopelessness or despair or, more simply, as essential aspects of an enriched, textured analytic relationship.

Transference as an Opportunity for Insight and Ensuing Structural Change versus Transference as an Opportunity for Developmental Progression

Historical Perspective

The third aspect that we wish to consider in this process of reconceptualizing transference is development. Development was not conceptualized as a specific aspect of analytic process for some time in the history of the field. For example, in Freudian (1905) theory libidinal development, which served as the underpinning of all development in Freud's model, ends with the offset of adolescence, there being no concept of ongoing development in adulthood. Freud explained pathology as the adult patient's having been unable successfully to resolve the Oedipus complex in childhood, leading to defensive fixation on the oedipal level, or to regression to phallic, anal, or oral levels of libidinal progression, interrupting thereby healthy, adequate movement into latency and through adolescence. Analysis served to resolve, via interpretation and working through in the transference, the unconscious conflicts that had interrupted normal development during the patient's childhood. Once that conflict was resolved, a libidinal phase progression could take place, with alterations and strengthening of psychic structure occurring in the patient in the context of the analytic process. However, this was not conceptualized as development per se, because, by definition, the adult is fully developed, inhibited as he or she may be by certain libidinal (and aggressive) phase fixations. Hence, any change for the better in adult life must be thought of in different terms, for example, as conflict resolution, more adaptive defenses, or alteration of the superego toward more realistic standards and criteria for guilt and shame. This tradition of viewing development as ceasing with the offset of adolescence has continued in classical analysis to the present, with development in the adult even now not incorporated in classical analytic theory (e.g., Brenner, 1982; Tyson & Tyson, 1990). In fact, in most analytic frameworks the adult patient undergoing developmental changes in an analytic process is not within the realm of consideration.

An alternative strategy was made possible only when Erik Erikson (1950) postulated that development occurs in adulthood, creating conceptual space for the model of adult analysis as a developmental experience. But it was Hans Loewald (1960) who placed it most forcefully and directly into analytic process, noting that the analytic relationship between patient and analyst had the effect of raising the patient to the developmental level of the analyst. This was prefigured by James Strachey (1934) in an important paper on developmental changes in the superego related to the analyst's participation in the relationship. William Meissner (1991) conceptualizes this developmental aspect of adult analysis as taking place within the therapeutic alliance. Moreover, many child analysts, following Loewald, have been attuned to the developmental impact for the adult patient of the analytic relationship (e.g., Coper on child analysis, in Goodman, 1977; M. Shane 1977; Settledge, Curtis, Lozoff, Siberschatz, & Simberg, 1988).

A more recent trend has been to conceptualize adult development as occurring specifically in the transference, actually conflated with it. For example, Kohut (1984) includes development as an important aspect of selfobject function. We believe that his original description of narcissistic gratifications in the analysis, which he termed "transference-like" experiences, were meant to convey that, in the process of experiencing with the analyst longings based on unfulfilled developmental needs, a new "corrective emotional experience" ensues within the analytic relationship which has developmental effect. At the same time, other self psychologists (e.g., Goldberg, 1978, 1990) specifically claim for the selfobject transference not a developmental impact, but instead, through the patient's experience of the optimally frustrated transference longing being understood by the analyst via interpretation, the patient achieves insight and structural change, a process akin to that observed in the classical analytic model (though the form of the transference and the content of the interpretation differs markedly).

Stolorow et al. (1987) brought development into the transference in a way that clarified Kohut's understanding. One pole of the bipolar transference they conceptualize, termed the selfobject-developmental pole, addresses the Kohutian insight of adult development ensuing through the selfobject functions of the analyst. In Stolorow et al.'s model, then, the developmental aspect of analysis is included, with transference being expanded to encompass this adult developmental experience under its rubric.

In summary, we identify three models for the relationship between transference and development. In the first, development is not conceptualized as occurring in the adult at all, and therefore there is no place within the analytic framework for developmental experience in the adult patient, and hence no confusion of development with transference. In the second, development in the adult is conceptualized in the analytic framework and does take place within the analysis, but it is conceptualized as occurring mainly in the therapeutic alliance sector of the relationship, which includes both the positive unobjectionable transference and the real relationship. However, because the therapeutic alliance concept is interwoven with the concept of transference, confusion of development with transference does ensue. In the third model, development in the adult patient is conceptualized as taking place within an aspect of the transference, so that transference and development are deliberately conflated. In one model, then, adult development is not conceptualized, and in the other two, it is a conflated concept, conflated either with the therapeutic alliance, or with the transference, or with both.

Developmental Systems Self Psychology Perspective

In our model, development is a centrally important concept, but we do not include it in our circumscribed definition of transference. To the contrary, our assumption is that in the relational configuration we describe as transference, the old self with old other relational configuration, the patient cannot develop, but instead exists in an arrested, suspended, repetitive state, where self-protective patterns arising in a relationship between the traumatized self and the traumatogenic other were the best means of sustaining the self and maintaining the tie to the other, with the cost to the self that development could not proceed.

Further, our assumption is that the analytic process itself is ultimately one of developmental progression; the relational configurations, which, ideally, move from the transference (old–old) into the old–new and new–new relational patterns, represent an important aspect of that developmental progression, a trajectory that is seen to move, on a macrolevel, configured in a linear fashion, toward the attainment of a healthy consolidation of the self and a healthy consolidation of the tie to the other. On a microlevel such a forward direction may not be apparent because what is visualized and experienced on that level appears disorganized, without visible pattern or trajectory (Thelen & Smith, 1994), or may even temporarily move in the opposite direction, toward or into old–old.

In the view put forward in this model, development is conceptualized as progression toward the attainment of a consolidation of the self and a consolidation of the intimate tie with the other. A healthy self depends on these capacities, and these capacities in turn are based on a foundation of secure attachment. We further maintain that insecure attachment patterns represent development gone awry, because these attachment patterns do not provide the secure base we posit as necessary to facilitate the attainment of either a consolidated self or a consolidated intimate tie with the other. In this postulate, we depart from the position of many attachment researchers who do not, as we do, categorize insecure attachment as skewed development. Although we do agree that such forms of attachment may very well represent the best, or only, available alternative for the infant during the first year of life and thereafter, they nevertheless compromise consolidation of self and tie to other. Ainsworth (1985), for example, writes that it is in response to the cues signaled by the mother that the infant's pattern of attachment is selected as the form that will most effectively permit closeness to the attachment figure. Although we agree that this would seem to be the best the infant can do under the circumstances, we contend that the emergence of an insecure attachment pattern is self-protective, and that such a choice made of necessity does not serve the infant in later life as well as a secure attachment might. A secure attachment allows for flexibility and choice, whereas an insecure attachment does not. Some attachment theorists assert that for some children, a secure attachment is not the most adaptive. For a child living in a violent neighborhood or an abusive home, for example, they maintain it is neither helpful nor adaptive for the therapist to strive to create a secure pattern of attachment with that child. The reasoning is that an open, trusting form of relatedness is not protective in dangerous situations. We disagree with this reasoning. If one understands secure attachment to include self-reflective capacities, as well as flexibility in accommodation and assimilation, then an environmentally endangered child who has a secure attachment relationship can reflect on the safest strategy and most self-protective form of attachment for the situation at hand. Should avoidance be reasoned by the child to be the safest option, for example, the child could then draw on this approach as the best choice given the circumstances.

Research conducted by Fonagy and his colleagues (Fonagy, Steele, Steele, Moran, & Higgitt, 1991) supports our view that secure attachment is the only attachment that has developmental potential inherent in it. On the basis of his findings, Fonagy speculates that when the infant is not able to anticipate that caregivers will respond accurately to his or her needs, the infant's response is to develop defensive strategies, or, in our terms, self-protective strategies, which in turn ultimately interfere with the achievement of the self-reflective capacity in the developing child, and hence with the achievement of a consolidated self. Insecure attachment results.

In further and more extended support of our position, we will include at this point several important quotations from the work of L. Alan Sroufe (1996) to support this significant and controversial aspect of our framework. Sroufe has conducted an ongoing longitudinal study of 180 children and their families, begun in 1974 and following the subjects year by year from their birth to their early adulthood. Sroufe, in describing the extreme importance of secure attachment, states the following:

> The effective dyadic regulation of emotion in infancy (secure attachment) is predicted to have consequences for emerging expectations concerning emotional arousal, and, at the behavioral level, consequences for the expression, modulation, and flexible control of emotions by the child. Those infants participating in a smoothly functioning, well-regulated relationship have repeatedly experienced: (1) That others are available and respond when they are emotionally aroused, (2) that emotional arousal is rarely disorganizing, and (3) that should such arousal be disorganizing, restabilization commonly is quickly achieved. Based on such expectations, children with secure attachment histories should readily engage situations having the potential for emotional arousal, and should directly express emotions, since emotions themselves are not threatening and are expected to be treated as communications by others. Thus, children with histories of secure attachment would be predicted to exhibit a notable curiosity, a zest for exploration, and affective expressiveness, especially in social situations. Likewise, when even strong affect is aroused, these children typically should remain organized, should manifest efforts to modulate arousal, and should effectively turn to others if their own capacities fail. They should be emotionally flexible or "resilient" . . . with the expression of impulses and emotion varying with context (e.g., exuberant on the playground, contained during reading time), and with the capacity to rebound following experiences of high threat and/or emotional arousal. (p. 189)

Here Sroufe (1996) has taken us through his sample population with predictions drawn from secure attachment and insecure attachment in infancy into the school years, predictions that are strongly supported by the research he presents. His research demonstrates the positive effects of secure attachment history over the lifespan from infancy into adulthood with children functioning into later childhood

"with aspects of competence, such as curiosity, self-esteem, independence, . . . positive peer behavior, [and] self-regulation" (p. 210).
Sroufe adds that children who are securely attached enjoy being with
others and show concern and regard for their welfare. "They were
nurturant with less able partners, and self-assertive with aggressive
partners. . . . Valuing themselves they will not tolerate exploitation;
caring for others they do not exploit" (p. 226).

This picture of securely attached children drawn from Sroufe's
research through early adulthood contrasts markedly with the picture
he draws of children who are insecurely attached and how they
mature. In the same study referred to above, Sroufe (1996) describes
infants who are insecurely attached, a predictable response, he says,
to unavailable or inconsistently available care. He notes that in the
ambivalent and avoidant attachment groups two possible strategies
for adaptation arise. In the case of the ambivalently attached child,
the child treats a wide array of situations as threatening, perpetually
appealing to the caregiver and/or seeking continual contact. In the
case of the avoidantly attached child, the child cuts himself or
herself off from affective experience, especially the need for tender
care.

Sroufe does not address the third category of insecure attachment identified by Mary Main (e.g., Main & Hesse, 1992), disorganized attachment. Main's research demonstrates that these children,
Category D disorganized attachment children, in response to fright
and helplessness engendered by the caregiver who is both feared and
needed, show approach behavior alternated with freezing, playing
dead, or other unusual or bizarre manifestations. Main and Hesse
(1992) correlate these manifestations with later dissociative defenses.
Although these authors may not specifically regard the bizarre-
appearing behavior as strategies per se taken to protect the self from
impending danger, our clinical experience would lead us to consider
these early attempts at dissociation as consistent and coherent strategies serving to screen out painful experience. This notion is supported by the research of Mary Sue Moore (1994). Although Sroufe
(1996) does not consider Category D babies and children as part of
his research, nevertheless his findings are consistent with other research and conceptions regarding such insecurely attached individuals.

Sroufe follows his observations on infants who are insecurely
attached with these comments on their later childhood development:

They are vulnerable to low self-esteem and a sense of incompetence, with associated feelings of worthlessness, guilt, and depression. Defenses, which can normally serve young children, can become engrained defensive strategies. Some children are characteristically (1) easily frustrated, overstimulated, tense, and anxious; (2) dependent, passive, and helpless; (3) hostile, aggressive, and anti-social; (4) emotionally insulated; or (5) profoundly disconnected from experience. The first two of these, reminiscent of resistant attachment, are defensive in postponing actual autonomous coping, in calling for continual adult care. The latter three serve to keep people and feelings at a distance. All tend to foreclose on the development of flexible strategies of emotional regulation. (1996, p. 222)

Finally, youngsters who have a history of insecure attachment have difficulties with peer relationships: "Those with avoidant histories were often emotionally distant from or hostile toward other children. . . . In response to another's distress, they were significantly more likely to do that which would further distress the child" (Sroufe, 1996, pp. 226–227). Those with resistant histories tended to "hover on the fringes of a group, or engage only to retreat when upset. . . . They were perfect fodder for the bullying child, always becoming upset when targeted and never taking firm or effective action. In fact those with avoidant histories exploited only children with resistant histories, or another avoidant child who had some special vulnerability" (p. 227).

We would like to mention briefly here the course of development with Category D infants as is revealed in other research studies. van der Kolk, McFarlane, and Weisaeth (1996), Herman (1992), and Davies and Frawley (1994) all describe individuals who are included in this Category D of attachment as developing a vulnerability to self-regulatory difficulties, to posttraumatic stress disorder, self-fragmentation, and repeated victimization.

We have spent this amount of time on Sroufe's (1996) and others' research concerning longitudinal effects of attachment categories on the developmental course of the individual for several reasons. First, we make a clinical assumption that attachment is of great importance developmentally, securing not only the tie to the other but consolidation of the self, as well. Second, and more specifically, we include this experimental work of others here to support our contention—which is, after all, different from that postulated by many attachment researchers—that insecure attachment is not just a variant of normal, but, in our perspective, represents an inflexible relational pattern that over the course of time becomes maladaptive. Third, and most relevant to our work, we conceptualize all disorders of the self as based in trauma, and we contend that these disorders are connected in a bidirectional fashion to insecure (traumatic) attachment patterns. As we have indicated, we can and do agree that it may very well represent for the infant or growing child the best or only adaptive strategy available to protect the self and the attachment tie, but even here, we believe that, were there some way to attain a secure attachment from another source, this would have served better the insecurely attached population even in coping with the tie to the primary caregiver. In this we are in agreement with Kohut (1977), who notes the importance of compensatory structure developed in the selfobject surround when the primary caretakers fail. We are also in agreement with Bowlby who notes that secure attachment with other than the primary caretakers can improve the attachment pattern of the insecurely attached individual toward a more secure attachment, and/or may make available a new, secure one. These latter views pertain to the importance in the analytic relationship of the new attachment to the analyst, which we will discuss below, and also point to one significant assumption inherent in our model, that is, our contention that analysis is best conducted in an atmosphere of positive ambience wherein the patient's safety and security are kept as central features, and wherein the analyst strives to respond to the patient's needs in whatever ways may be helpful to the patient's development consistent with the analyst's capacities and limitations. In this atmosphere, we believe, progression in analysis can take place.

At this point we would add a caveat to our discussion of development within the analytic relationship. It is widely argued that psychoanalysts tend to extrapolate unjustifiably both from infancy to adulthood, infantomorphizing the adult, and, often, from adulthood to infancy, as well, adultomorphizing the infant. It is contended further that analysts in so doing disregard the significant differences between these two levels of development in order to emphasize the proposed similarities. We obviously can be accused of doing this very thing, of drawing too directly from infancy research to understand the adult analytic situation. In our own defense, we can argue that of course we do not consider the analyst–patient relationship as identical to the parent–child relationship. We use the parent–child attachment patterns in part as metaphor for understanding patterns of relatedness in the analytic dyad and to guide and constrain our clinical efforts. But the data quoted above, as well as other data we consider elsewhere in this book, would indicate a connection that goes beyond metaphor. We believe that self- and mutual-regulatory processes, affect attunement, self-reflective capacities, self-protective strategies, as well as categories of attachment, are directly active in the adult and in adult–adult relationships, just as they are throughout childhood. These connections between childhood and adulthood are experimentally traceable in a linear fashion to manifestations in the clinical world. We are impressed that securely attached individuals on the whole function more effectively in the world throughout the discernible life cycle, and that secure attachment is the basis for that consolidation of the self and consolidation of the tie to the other that we connect to emotional health. It is this very process of securing a consolidated attachment tie and a concomitant consolidation of self that we believe constitutes development in the analytic relationship, with all of the capacities that are inherent in these attainments. To review, capacities of a consolidated self include those that constitute an integrated self, Stern's (1985) concepts of affectivity, historicity, agency, and self-cohesion. In addition, the consolidated self in our model encompasses a capacity for full intersubjective awareness and sharing; a robust sense of reality; a heightened self-reflective attainment; and abilities for pleasure, intimacy, adaptive self-protection, and creativity.

In sum, we believe that if an analytic procedure or stance could somehow facilitate this kind of development in the analytic relationship, meliorative change would occur, the kind of change sought by every analyst within every analytic framework. The challenge lies in a central question: Can such a significant and far-reaching development take place in an adult or a child through the analytic experience itself, based on understanding, insight, and a living-through relationship with the analyst? We believe it can. However, such a bold accomplishment requires specific attributes both in the analyst and in the milieu that he or she co-creates with the patient. The analyst should respond to the patient, we contend, in the way in which someone responds who has himself or herself been securely attached and who wants to secure that experience for another. Availability, concern, positive responsiveness, positive regard, a commitment to the patient's well-being, and an encouraging attitude in regard to all the patient's struggles and conflicts, as well as wishes and desires, these all appear in the analytic attitude that pertains in our model, promoting, we believe, the kind of development we have described.

Relational Configurations and the Trajectory of Developmental Progression

THE RELATIONAL CONFIGURATIONS: THE PATIENT'S PERSPECTIVE

In the previous chapter we introduced our effort to reconceptualize transference, indicating that, in our own model, transference is conceptualized as but one of the three relational configurations we identify as evolving in the analytic situation. These three relational configurations, describing an aspect of the connection between patient and analyst, are organized in terms of the trajectory of developmental progression that we see as an important component of forward movement in development in general, and in analysis in particular, a movement toward consolidation of the self and consolidation of the intimate tie to the other. As such, the configurations describe, as we indicated earlier, a continuum from old to new, from childhood to adulthood, from suffering to health, or, to paraphrase Robert Stoller (1975), from trauma to triumph.

We will outline the relational configurations in more detail shortly, but listed briefly, they are, first, the *old self with old other patient–analyst relational configuration*, in which the patient currently experiences both self and analyst in a repetition of patterns categorized predominantly on the basis of traumatic past lived experience, patterns that encompass the old, traumatized self with the old, traumatogenic other; second, the *old self with new other patient–analyst relational configuration*, in which the patient continues to categorize himself or herself predominantly in old, traumatized ways but is beginning to experience the analyst as different from traumatogenic figures in the past; and third, the *new self with new other patient–analyst relational configuration*, in which the patient categorizes both himself or herself and the analyst predominantly in positive new ways not based on the traumatogenic past. Although we recognize that memory, being best understood as the recategorization of experience, ensures that there are always elements of the past recategorized in the present, in this last relational configuration there is predominance of current, novel, in-the-moment perception and experience, in contrast to past perception and experience. This complex recategorization process defining the patient's experience of self and analyst in the moment is understood intersubjectively and interpersonally as positive new happenings between the two persons in the room at the present time rather than as relivings from the traumatic past.

Several important points follow:

1. Out of the numerous configurations one might conceivably identify, we choose to identify these three categories of relational configuration because they are, from our perspective, the most pertinent configurations in tracking the developmental trajectory that leads toward consolidation of the self and consolidation of the intimate tie to the other.

2. We describe here these three configurations as taken from the *patient's* perspective; later in this chapter we describe the same configurations as taken from the *analyst's* perspective. The nature of the analyst's experience of the relational configuration may be quite different from that of the patient; hence, for didactic purposes, the analyst's relational pattern must be considered separately, though of course both perspectives operate simultaneously and interrelatedly in the analytic situation, mutually influencing one another in the clinical, selfother system. However, as one might expect in such a heuristic classification, these configurations may not be experienced in pure form, but often overlap.

3. We emphasize the "traumatogenic," defining that concept broadly, because in our model analysis is concerned with the alleviation of pain and suffering, which we contend emerges primarily as a result of unmastered, painful, lived experience, that is, from trauma.

4. We do not mean to say that old relationships cannot be facilitative, nor that positive old relationships are insignificant, nor that they do not have a part in the analytic investigation. We have

already indicated our view of the role of positive old relationships that have been adequately assimilated and accommodated to by the patient. We oppose the role of such positive experiences with the role of those more negative, traumatic experiences that have been sequestered from such ongoing accommodation. The latter remain fixed and inflexible, so that the painful past continues to be brought into the new present, resulting in current experience being assimilated into past traumatic patterns. Through the three relational configurations we have delineated, we describe aspects of the trajectory of developmental progression, which constitutes an important component of developmental change.

5. A given relational configuration is co-constructed by patient and analyst. Although the configuration as described represents the analyst's distillation of the patient's experience of the relationship at any given time, how the configuration itself is understood is based on what patient and analyst have contributed and constructed together in the dyad, keeping in mind that the constellation is heavily informed by the person of the analyst and his or her theories, along with who the patient is and what the patient has experienced in the past.

6. From a systems perspective, we are describing with these three relational configurations a phenomenon analogous to what Thelan and Smith (1994) have termed *attractor states*. By borrowing this concept we hope to facilitate understanding of how relational configurations in the analytic dyad change. Thelan and Smith note that attractor states in the individual appear stable enough to take on the characteristics of permanent structure, but when looked at more closely and in more detail, these attractor states appear "soft assembled," meaning that under certain conditions they can be dissolved. These authors describe how change occurs in the individual: With sufficient perturbation, a particular attractor state, such as an individual's fear-laden, dread-infused quality of relatedness to others, which can appear invariant, can be reconfigured into a different attractor state, or quality of relatedness, of trustful safety in connection with others. Using this as a model for change, an aspect of analytic work within a particular relational configuration can be viewed as a means to perturb the patient–analyst system such that new, more currently adaptive developmentally advanced states are attained and maintained. That is, the work of analysis is to determine how the relationship between patient and analyst can be altered from an old pattern in which the analyst is viewed as a traumatogenic other and the self as the traumatized self, to a new pattern in which the analyst is

perceived as a new, helpful other, both self-transforming and interpersonal intimacy sharing, and the self moves toward a more adaptive consolidation.

Below, we elaborate the patterns themselves.

The Old Self with Old Other
Patient–Analyst Relational Configuration

Here we will review important aspects of this configuration that have been articulated previously in our discussion of reconceptualizing transference, placing these aspects now within the perspective of a fuller description of the old self with old other patient–analyst relational configuration. By this pattern we refer to a current relationship with the analyst wherein both the analyst and the self are perceived by the patient, with or without self-reflection, as figures predominantly organized on the basis of traumatic relational experiences with significant, traumatogenic others from the past. We conceptualize trauma broadly as including experiences of loss, deprivation, intrusion, or neglect, as well as threatened, perceived, or actual danger to the physical well-being of the self. Such experiences may occur over a period of time, or may constitute short-term or even single episodes; the defining features are the sense of helplessness and of being overwhelmed, accompanied by other dysphoric affects and bodily experiences, and leading to the sequestering of aspects of the self. Such sequestering strategies, which we conceptualize as self-protective, are invoked to attempt mastery of the trauma and to defend against future trauma. The patient's ensuing relationship patterns tend to remain fixed and inflexible as ways of being with an other that had been experienced as relatively adaptive at some time in the past, as the best or only way available to the individual under traumatic circumstances, which no longer pertain in the present. Simply put, the analyst is assimilated, either consciously or unconsciously, into the old, familiar pattern, self in interaction with important, potentially traumatic other, possibly the only pattern as yet available to the patient, or, alternatively, the only pattern that can be safely allowed in the present. Moreover, the patient's assimilation of the analyst may either take the form of a repetition of the original role relationship, or take the form of a role reversal, with the self as other, and the other as self. Our old self with old other patient–analyst relational configuration, then, is akin to the transference configuration well described and ubiquitous in analytic literature, referred to, for example, as the *transference neurosis* in the classical literature (Freud, 1912; Greenson, 1967), the *iconic transference* of Modell (1988), the *archaic failed selfobject transference* in self psychology (Kohut, 1971), and the *repetitive conflictual pole of the transference* in intersubjectivity theory (Stolorow et al., 1987). Again we emphasize that we limit the term "transference" to this particular relational configuration.

The Old Self with New Other
Patient–Analyst Relational Configuration

By this pattern we refer to a current analytic relationship wherein the patient continues to feel caught in old, traumatized ways, incapable of feeling differently about himself or herself, but nevertheless is beginning to experience the analyst as a person different from past, traumatizing others, a novel other, one without prototype in the patient's life, not categorized predominantly on unassimilated conscious, preconscious, or defensively sequestered (unconscious) patterns from the past. The analyst may appear, for example, as soothing, comforting, understanding, regulating, and insight providing, or as one who is able to be and to remain with the patient in painful and frightening experiences. However, the patient continues, as in the past, to suffer from these painful experiences and to view himself or herself in a dysphoric manner. This relational configuration represents a transitional shift from an old self with old other, on the way to a new self with new other patient–analyst relational configuration, but this transitional position may persist in the analysis for a long time. Moreover, the configuration may alter in either direction so that the pattern in the analysis may revert to an old self with old other patient–analyst relational configuration rather than move forward in the developmental trajectory.

The New Self with New Other
Patient–Analyst Relational Configuration

By this pattern we refer to an analytic relationship describing the patient's emergent achievement of a balance between accommodation and assimilation, a balanced equilibration, a developing capacity for organizing current experiences of self and self with other in new and different ways instead of persistently organizing self and self with other based on a recategorization predominantly influenced by traumatogenic experience from the past. The new self is an integrated self, with affectivity, agency, historicity, and coherence; moreover, the new self is a consolidated self, with capacities for intersubjective and interpersonal relatedness, for mature self-reflective awareness, with a solidly endowed sense of reality, capacities for pleasure and intimacy, and the ability for invoking creative self-elaborative and adaptive self-protective strategies that do not disrupt the self's consolidation. This integrated and consolidated self has been attained in the analysis through positive new experiences with the analyst as a novel other so that a consolidated, secure tie to the analyst has been achieved in the analytic ambience of safety, comfort, and intimacy sharing.

THE TRAJECTORY OF DEVELOPMENTAL PROGRESSION

Moving now to the trajectory of developmental progression as it applies to the relational configurations we have identified, we want to make the point first that the relational configuration that emerges at any given time in the analysis cannot be predicted in a linear fashion, nor can these relational configurations be predicted with absolute certainty on the basis of particular analytic interventions. We can cite, however, actions of the analyst that may lead to either development-inducing or development-impeding patterns in each of the three configurations we have identified.

In terms of the old self with old other patient–analyst relational configuration (old–old), it is development-inducing for patient and analyst to be immersed together in the repetition of important traumatic experiences from the past where those experiences are retained as unconsciously sequestered or otherwise defended against, where they are preconsciously or unconsciously feared and/or sought out for purposes of connection or mastery, or where, more simply, there is no other way available to the patient in which the experience can be organized. In any of these cases, the traumatic experiences are inaccessible to reorganization through positive new experience. That is, the old–old configuration is the only way that the patient can relate, but such a connection in the dyad will hopefully allow for the eventual recognition, interpretation, and understanding of the patient's past traumatic experience. After all, it is through such interactions that the patient's self is consolidated, with self-understanding, self-reflective capacities, self- and mutual regulation, and the like being enhanced.

This is what we mean when we say that the trajectory of developmental progression is in process, and that though the relational configuration remains for the most part caught in old–old, there is nevertheless movement within the old–old relationship of the kind just described, but with positive new experience in connection with the analyst either still unattainable for the patient or not as yet evident in the process. An example follows:

An artist patient referred for analysis presented with such disorganization that the analyst, puzzled by the degree of her fragmented and disordered thought, considered a diagnosis of organic brain dysfunction. As it turned out, that diagnosis was accurate, but based on chemical addiction. The patient revealed that she had for many years used marijuana a minimum of twice a day. Patient and analyst began by attempting to reduce the marijuana intake, and gradually, through this reduction, the unbearable affects of deadness, absence of vitality, and lack of motivation, as well as suicidal self states became apparent, and the efforts at self-medication became clear. As the analyst slowly began to replace the medication with her own person, as a self-transforming other, providing the self-regulation, soothing, and containing the patient so desperately needed, it became possible as well to come in touch with the traumatic experiences that had been the patient's lifelong legacy. An old–old relational configuration emerged and remained in play, off and on, for several years. The patient felt, for the most part, despair and blackness, with the analyst unable to be taken in at all as a new person who could be helpful. The patient felt alone in the office, in the same way that she had, so much of the time, been alone in her bedroom at home, and alone as well even in her parents' presence.

Her parents had been and remained throughout treatment self-preoccupied and essentially nonresponsive to their child's needs. Although they agreed to keep her in treatment, they were willing to pay only a minimum fee, despite the fact that they had considerable means at their disposal.

The old–old pattern arising in the treatment proved essential to patient and analyst in order to allow for the old self states and the old unbearable affects to emerge, be clarified, and be lived through. These states had been sequestered and had remained unconscious, though they obviously strongly influenced the patient's day-to-day experience and functioning, along with her resorting to self-medication in an effort to reduce her psychological pain. In treatment the affect states could be observed and articulated, making sense for the patient of her experience of empty depression. This took time, requiring the maintenance of an old–old pattern until sufficient understanding and regulation could be achieved. A marker of progress was the change in the patient's artwork and in her dress over a period of time.

Once the analysis had begun and access was gained by the patient to her heretofore sequestered traumatic states, the patient began to paint at home abstract patterns heavily dominated by black hues in order to regulate, express, and cope with her feelings, and then to bring these paintings into the sessions for the analyst's perusal. At the same time she began to wear only black clothing. She had to stay in that darkness until her moods and their multiple sources were shared and clarified. Only then did her paintings begin to take on color, and only then did she allow color in her clothing. Our point here is that the analyst understood the necessity to uncover old traumatic experience for this patient in the old–old connection for so long as these affects and moods remained sequestered and disavowed. As the dissociation was reduced, and the sequestering eliminated, the memories and feelings could be integrated into the self, making room for both a coherent self-narrative and for a developmental progression to old–new, and then, eventually, to new–new in the movement toward self- and self-with-other consolidation. Hence the old–old relational configuration had proved facilitative of development with this patient, and progression in the analysis was marked by movement within that old–old pattern.

The old–old relational configuration is *not* facilitative of development when further immersion is deemed unnecessary because there has already been sufficient recognition, interpretation, understanding, and integration of the old traumatic experience as repeated in the relationship. At some point in time—a point that is obviously impossible to predict, but that can be perceived by the analyst, either consciously or unconsciously, on the basis of a myriad of factors, through planning or serendipitously, and always in the form of trial and error amid the unformulated stream of lived experience, going mainly on clinical feel based on the guidelines and values we are attempting to articulate—the analyst does something. That is, the analyst makes a move that reveals him or her to be different from figures in the patient's past, and the patient this time, for whatever reason, can appreciate that difference. For example, the analyst may offer an extra appointment at a time of mutually perceived need, or may offer to call while on vacation, and the patient can accept the offer on the terms it is made. Or the patient may at some point take the initiative, with a declaration or series of declarations familiar to all clinicians: "This is not helpful," "I know all of this already," "It's all the same old thing over and over," "Now what?"

We contend that the reliving of pain *for its own sake* is not useful, and in and of itself does not lead to developmental change. Where interpretation, understanding, and integration have, ostensibly, done their work, the patient benefits from something new. Examples of this counterproductive perseveration in an old–old relational configuration are found most clearly, often in dramatic form, with patients who have experienced such severe trauma that they are the victims of flashback phenomena or other forms of traumatic reliving. In such cases, this overemphasis on the old–old relational configuration, or too much or too rapid exposure or uncovering within such a configuration, without attention to the support of the self and to the provision of safety, can lead to the patient's self-fragmentation, experience of flooding, or further self-protective retreat into dangerous and deleterious self states. The specifics of these interventions must be seen in context, as in the following example where the analyst had erred in inadvertently persisting in keeping her patient too long in an old–old relational configuration.

A young adolescent girl who suffered from cerebral palsy entered into analysis because of her unhappiness and depression ostensibly concerning her father's absence in her life. Her parents had divorced when she was very small, her mother had remarried, and her father was only available intermittently. None of this was new, yet her mother and stepfather could find no other reason for her obvious unhappiness in the present. The analyst was surprised to discover when she met her new patient the extent to which the girl suffered from involuntary movements of her limbs, not having been sufficiently prepared by the parents for an obvious handicap in their daughter. It became clear in a short time that there was another reason for her current depression: She had entered a new school and her peers were reacting to her as if she were different, in fact, a freak, whereas she herself had long ago stopped allowing her handicap to be her defining feature. She had the experience that once people had gotten to know her, the handicap disappeared as a consideration in her relationships. In time, analyst and patient understood how this current experience was different. Boys had entered the picture, and dating became an issue. What she had not allowed herself to face was the question, Would she ever have normal relationships with boys, and how would that happen?

This situation was explored for a period of time, during which, initially, the analyst was perceived by the patient as a new and helpful other in her life, one who could teach her about what to expect from boy-girl relationships. The patient herself had remained in an old self state, revisiting the times when she was younger and she was forced once again to recognize the existence of her handicap. This had happened each time she entered a new environment, and remained the case until she and the others got used to one another. All of this became clear and the treatment seemed to be going well, but then slowly and inexplicably the patient began to express anger and discomfort with the analyst, and showed a new stubborn reluctance to talk to her. The analyst was puzzled and confused about this behavior; on the outside it seemed her patient was doing better in school and with her peers, yet she seemed progressively more unhappy in the analysis.

Finally it was the patient herself who explained the situation. She said that she was tired of her analyst seeing her as disabled, that she had expected her analyst to be able, like others had done before, to see her as a whole person, not just as one who has shakes and trembles. The analyst on her part realized that she had been inadvertently retraumatizing the patient, keeping her in an old–old configuration beyond its usefulness in understanding what the patient had originally brought into treatment. Fortunately, the patient had sufficient insight and self-reflection, and sufficient trust in the analyst, to clarify the situation, and the analyst was able to see the patient differently, as no longer currently traumatized by her disability. They could turn to a more productive exploration of the patient's experiences with her new peers and in her new phase of life, with an emergence of a new–new relational configuration.

We also want to stress that from our perspective it is destructive for the analyst to seek out old–old configurations for their own sake, or on the basis of theory, for example, on the basis of the postulate that without a direct revival in the relationship with the analyst of dysphoric affect and traumatic repetitions from the past, nothing is really happening in the analytic work. For example, a patient who was attacked murderously by her psychotic mother as a child saw her analyst as a safe harbor, but she experienced with her own child a sudden impulse to seriously harm the child, justified in her own mind as consequent to the child's extreme and defiant misbehavior. With her child, then, and not with her analyst, the patient confronted directly and with powerful affect painful experiences stemming from her past. Then, coming in and using her analyst as a background of safety and a secure base, she was able to connect the experience with her child with her own past trauma, via role reversal, she having taken the role of her mother vis-à-vis her child, who was in the role of herself. We believe, then, that it is possible successfully to relive trauma by turning passive into active with another person outside the analytic dyad, and that it is not always necessary to do so directly and dramatically with the analyst. In our view, in fact, a persistent attempt to get a patient to reexperience the trauma directly with the analyst— in this case, for example, by interpreting the anger as a defensive displacement of feelings that are actually experienced in the transfer-ence relationship—might represent a traumatic invalidation of the patient's powerfully lived experience with her child, creating iatro-genic pathology in its own right. In this last example, we see an old self with old other relational configuration enacted in reverse outside of the analysis, and an old self with new other patient–analyst rela-tional configuration examined within the context of the analytic relationship. That is, the patient, in an old, traumatized state, feared she had done damage to her child, and might do further damage in that same state, but felt hopeful at the same time that the analyst, experienced as a new other, could help her in positive new ways.

This leads us into a consideration of the trajectory of develop-mental progression as it relates to our second relational configuration, the old–new. Here what evidences developmental progression is the emergence in the patient's experience of the analyst as a new other, as in the example cited above, distinguishable from a continuation or revival of relatedness with old, traumatizing figures from the past. It is only this enhanced capacity in the patient to perceive the other, the analyst, as unique and different that allows the pair to experience and articulate the genetic and present-day contributions to the pa-tient's dysphoria as derivative from and continuous with self states and relational patterns from the past. Only when this traumatized self state can be understood in the context of a positive new experience with the other in the present is there potential for a new self state to evolve, encompassing a capacity for self-consolidation with all the develop-mental concomitants we have identified, moving the patient along the trajectory on the way to the co-creation of a new self with new other patient–analyst relational configuration. Hence it is particularly in this context that the "new" in the old–new constellation represents the key meliorative element leading to the patient's developmental pro-gression within the analysis.

In contrast, the old–new relational configuration is *not* development inducing when it derives from the analyst's being unable or
unwilling to remain in the old–old relational configuration long
enough to allow for sufficient understanding of old relational patterns
from the past, when the analyst, that is, cannot refrain from prematurely introducing interventions that distract the patient in order to
avoid in either member of the dyad pain that cannot be tolerated by
the analyst. Movement from old–old to old–new is again *not* development inducing when the analyst cannot permit himself or herself to
stay with the patient's perceptions and expectations, but again prematurely explains his or her own part in an impasse that has arisen
between them, disrupting the patient's need to remain, along with the
analyst, immersed in the old–old for long enough to understand it and
to live it through. For example, an analyst, in the face of his impending
vacation and the patient's resultant terror, suggested that the patient
might be stronger than the patient knew and so might be able to get
through the vacation without so much difficulty. On his part, the
patient, hearing the analyst's comment, felt even more terror because
the analyst obviously could not understand the patient's inability as
yet to keep the analyst in mind when they were apart.

However, from the perspective of developmental progression,
immersion experiences in the old–new relational configuration are not
enough, either. For example, staying as the comforting, soothing, and
interpreting figure for the patient's traumatized state may become
static, and the patient may get the sense that the most one can hope
for in analysis is to be understood and attuned to in a state of misery.
The traditional analytic response at this point is either to insist that
not enough has been understood to make a difference or, alternatively,
to insist that the changes that would make a difference have to be
sought for and experienced by the patient outside of the analysis.
Although both, or either, of these contentions may at times be
accurate, we hold that the developmental trajectory must progress to
the point where a new–new relational configuration is experienced in
the analysis, one where the patient achieves with the analyst not only
a newly consolidated self, but a newly consolidated tie to the other,
providing thereby not only an experience for the patient of intimacy
sharing with the analyst, but also a new template or pattern that will
generate such relationships with others on the outside.

Failure to progress developmentally pertains in a premature effort
on the analyst's part to move the relationship into a new–new configuration, as well. This may happen when the analyst encourages too

soon or too hastily the patient's movement away from old–new toward new–new at the expense of remaining available in the old–new pattern, foreclosing the achievement of integrating all that can and must be learned there. For example, the analyst, in an attempt to restore with the patient a newly achieved positive experience, may remind that patient of a heretofore expressed, more hopeful mood and a more connected state, at a time when that patient feels the need to have the analyst remain immersed with him or her in an old, remembered dysphoric state attempting to achieve thereby a sense of not being alone in a traumatic state, and of being understood by a protective other in that state. By such premature pressure coming from the analyst, the patient is robbed of self-knowledge and of a sense of realness, as well as of a sense of the experience of a new other who can remain with him or her in unhappy times. Thus, the analyst's insistence, either conscious or unconscious, that the patient experience a new, positive perception of self in the analytic dyad is not in the service of developmental progression, that is, not in the service of the patient's authentic self-knowledge, solid integration, and a satisfying intimacy-sharing experience.

Finally, we contend that developmental progression in the patient requires that the analyst sustain the dimension of intimacy that appears most facilitative to the patient's overall trajectory. That is, the analyst must consider whether, in the particular relational configuration present in the foreground of the dyad, the analyst is perceived by the patient to be functioning as a self-transforming other or as an interpersonal-sharing other. We believe that it may not be development inducing, for example, for the patient who is deep into experiencing the analyst in the relationship primarily as a self-transforming other in an old–new relational configuration to be confronted by that analyst's misattuned attempt to achieve interpersonal sharing. On the other hand, it might hamper analytic progress for the analyst to refrain from introducing his or her own perspective when this perspective is judged to be potentially helpful to the patient, when, for example, the patient either needs that form of intimacy in old–new or seems to be moving into new–new and might benefit from an intimate connection with an interpersonal-sharing other. For example, an adolescent boy left his analyst of several years because that analyst had refused to share with him the kind of car the analyst drove. This refusal was experienced by the patient as an expression of the analyst's unwillingness to be in any personal connection with him, and he responded by feeling that the analyst was not someone to whom he himself wished to be connected.

We wish to clarify that we do not link either the old–new or the new–new relational configuration with a particular dimension of intimacy. That is, either the self-transforming or the interpersonal-sharing dimension, or both, can be present in old–new or new–new. Neither dimension of intimacy is present in old–old, as intimacy is not possible when the self is in a traumatic state with a traumatogenic other. Hence, the analyst must be sensitive both to the dimension of intimacy required by the patient, and to the relational configuration currently emergent in order best to induce the patient's development and to assure a positive new experience. All of these points will be illustrated in the clinical chapter that follows.

RECURRENT AND EMERGENT RELATIONAL CONFIGURATIONS IN THE CLINICAL FIELD FROM THE ANALYST'S PERSPECTIVE

We use the same three relational configurations we have already identified and described from the patient's perspective to address the view of the analytic dyad taken from the analyst's perspective, addressing that perspective as *analyst–patient,* rather than *patient–analyst* so as to clarify that the perspective has changed to that of the analyst. We believe that from the analyst's point of view, the relational configuration between analyst and patient ideally remains organized in the new self with new other, *analyst–patient* relational configuration as the baseline for effective analytic work. That is, the analyst, to function effectively as an analyst, must possess a consolidated self; must be able to consolidate a tie to an other; must be capable of establishing a bidirectional, self-transforming other connection to the patient; and, finally, must have capacities for interpersonal intimacy sharing. In turn, these abilities permit the analyst to decenter self-reflectively, viewing the patient clearly as a new individual, not conflated or confused with significant figures from the analyst's past, and viewing himself or herself also as new in that relationship. Again ideally, at times the analyst finds himself or herself dipping down into the past, either voluntarily or involuntarily—that is, either deliberately, in a search for experiences analogous to those of the patient, or spontaneously, stimulated by retrieval cues stemming from the current situation. At such times the analyst's capacity for self- and mutual reflection is either maintained or regained, allowing the analyst to self-right back into the new–new pattern, so much the wiser about self and/or patient for the visit into the old. Thus, new–new is that ideal, baseline relational configuration, taken from the analyst's perspective, that is most conducive to the patient's (and analyst's) ongoing development. Less ideally, the analyst may find himself or herself distracted by strategies of self-protection, such as self-preoccupations based on past experience, or the analyst may be distracted by visions of the patient as a revenant for the analyst of past, significant, traumatogenic others.

This leads us to a consideration of countertransference from a developmental systems self psychology perspective. We have said that the old–old relational configuration from the patient's perspective constitutes our definition of transference, akin to the transference neurosis, the archaic self–selfobject transference relationship, and the repetitive pole of the bipolar transference. In a parallel fashion, the old–old relational configuration from the analyst's perspective is our definition of countertransference, and is akin to the classical conception of countertransference, wherein both the self of the analyst and the self of the patient become assimilated by the analyst as figures from the past, that is, recategorized in terms of the analyst's old, traumatic relational configurations.

We will illustrate countertransference as it appears in our model with the following example. An analyst was treating two men, one, Bob G., in his middle 30s, the other, Albert F., slightly younger. Both were attorneys; both worked for the same large law firm, one being a partner and the other quite close to it; and both, as it turned out, discovered in time that they were in analysis with the same analyst.

Their reasons for coming to treatment were different, but the dimension of intimacy established with each was of an interpersonal-sharing variety. Bob, a tall, blonde, well-built man, had entered analysis first, about a year before Albert. He had just been made partner in his firm, and described as a principle concern his guilty response to a series of successes crowned by this latest achievement. He also suffered from obsessive doubting and a lack of pleasure in life. Bob was the youngest of five siblings in a family that included a brother and three sisters, a successful and tyrannically controlling father who had just died, and an overly protective and clinging mother made more so by the father's recent death. Bob's only brother had always been, without contest, the leader of the sibling family, the heir apparent of the family business, but he had suffered, a few years before, a severe accident that had created obvious emotional problems for him and subsequent interference with his business performance. These emotional difficulties prevented this brother from assuming the role the family had all anticipated for him, with Bob, the youngest and the coddled baby of the family, taking his older brother's place, in effect becoming both president of the family investment company and now partner in the large law firm. As Bob said of himself, things always came too easily to him, contributing to his obsessive fear of impending disaster, accentuating his guilty sense that he deserved disaster, and propelling him into analysis. As he and his analyst came to understand, the survival guilt Bob felt derived from a sense that he was taking from the others what was theirs; it was permitted for Bob to be preferred, but to be preferred and successful, too, meant to Bob that he was stealing his brother's share. Moreover, his sisters were neither preferred nor successful, adding to his guilt. This set of feelings interfered with Bob's capacity to allow himself a permanent relationship with a woman, another reason for seeking treatment and for choosing a woman analyst.

Bob saw himself immediately as the analyst's favorite. When he phoned her office for the first time asking for an appointment, he later reported that he could tell just from the way the analyst responded on the phone that she took an instant and irresistible liking to him. He felt she saw him as special and had made room for him in her busy practice when she did not really have the time available. Much of the content of the sessions right from the beginning was informed by a seductive, inviting, and charming effort to win the analyst's love, together with a feeling that it was his just for the asking. This view of himself was conceptualized by the analyst as reflecting the actual position he had always maintained in his family; it was not seen as a self-protective, entitled stance guarding him against feeling deprived, overlooked, and inferior. From the analyst's perspective, then, this was a patient who was not in need of a self-transforming experience. Instead, she felt responded to and recognized as a person in her own right, and reacted in turn by feeling an unusual interest in and receptivity toward him. She saw him as intelligent, handsome, and possessive of an ironic humor, with a capacity for an unusual self- and mutual reflection. In short, Bob was just very enjoyable, indeed pleasurable, for the analyst to work with, despite his doubting and unhappiness. The analyst reflected that she had to remain alert to her own erotically tinged attraction to her patient, and to wonder as well if he had indeed picked up some unusual interest in him. On reflection, she speculated that these unstated reactions on her part were more than likely making themselves known to him. Certainly Bob was ready to be seen as her favorite, which had made him perceive even the few words they exchanged in the original phone call as confirmation of her interest, but might there be something more in the analyst herself that was also ready to respond too receptively to him? What made Bob so appealing to her as a patient? Was it just that he was on the healthy end of the spectrum of her patient population? that he was able, and even happy, to pay her fee? that he got so much, so readily, from the analysis, improving at a better than average pace? She could not tell, but she knew she had to remain alert, that something out of her awareness might be astir in her to which her patient was responding.

Then, into the mix, came Albert, referred from a different source entirely, the son of a colleague from another city who was worried about Albert's depression and fearful that Albert was not advancing smoothly in life. According to his father, Albert had picked a girlfriend who had treated him badly, not valuing him sufficiently, and the father worried that Albert did not sufficiently value himself. Albert's view was different. He saw himself as having been, when he was young, the black sheep of his family, untidy, incorrigible, only average in school compared to his two brilliant siblings, and the only one among them who did not become a doctor as both of his parents were. Yet Albert felt that he was now the one preferred by his parents; both of his parents had artistic interests, and he himself was a talented writer who had chosen law as a profession relatively late, and only as a way of supporting himself. He wrote poetry and had published a novel in his 20s, which had given him a belated sense of winning the field, of being the chosen son. Although the analyst had known when he was first referred that Albert practiced in the same firm as her other patient, Bob, she knew also that the firm was very large, that Bob's and Albert's legal specialties and departments in the firm were different, and that it seemed likely that their paths would not ever cross. She took Albert into analysis, then, because she did not anticipate that her doing so would interfere with Bob's ongoing progress, imagining that it would not turn out to be a burden on either analysis.

Albert began his treatment by telling the analyst that although he anticipated that she would find him troublesome and untidy at first and would be critical of him for it, she would ultimately discover that he was lovable and very attractive, even sexually. He told her that his mother had certainly found him so, remembering some joking comment she had once made to her friend about what an irresistibly sexually attractive adolescent he had, against all odds, turned out to be. In fact, Albert had always had, despite his father's concerns, reasonably good relationships with women, and anticipated that in time the analyst would be another in the line of women who, like his mother, had reluctantly but somehow easily succumbed to his charms. And indeed, the analyst did find Albert to be of high interest to her. She, too, loved literature, had a background in poetry, and had as well a handsome son of about his age who was also a novelist, who had written his first book when he was 12, which he had dedicated to "my mother who loves to read."

As it turned out, much to the analyst's chagrin, the two patients did meet, and moreover, they came to spend many happy hours together discussing the analyst they shared, her faults, of course, but what she found more irresistible in the hearing, was that they talked a lot about her virtues, including their sense of her incredible sexual attractiveness. They saw her as fascinating, older to be sure, but still very desirable as a woman. They mused together about how much more attractive she must have been when she was younger. They told one another how they loved her, and playfully speculated as to whom between them she loved and desired most. They had lots of questions about her sexual life. All of this was repeated by each of them to her.

The analyst understood the genetic roots for their feelings and appreciated what was a positive new experience for each of them, of sharing openly with one another their emotions, a capacity novel for both and reflective of their progress in analysis. Each, that is, experienced a fun-filled attachment to a sibling, clearly a first for them both. They could enjoy a rivalry for the analyst without the guilt and fear over an anticipated victory of one over the other, as had been the fate for each of them in the past. The analyst, then, was clear about the meaning and importance of the experience for her patients. Moreover, she was not a novice in the treatment of attractive younger men who longed for a mutually sharing sexual intimacy with her, and who found her absorbing, possessing a mind capable of letting them know, and sharing with them things worth knowing. All of this was familiar enough, and she recognized a certain caution that was not new, either, but somehow the combination of two men who knew each other and who vied with each other for her attention was of more than ordinary interest to her and was hard to resist.

Despite herself she caught herself looking forward much more than usual to each of their hours and could not help but notice that she found herself somewhat disappointed when one or the other did not report that they had talked together about her. Of course it was troubling, especially this last, so she was careful, and insofar as she knew she attempted not to be too seductive, not to appear too interested in herself, and not to encourage the competition for her favor. She dealt with it in her usual fashion, trying to remain as introspectively aware as possible, keeping each patient's developmental needs in mind as she shared or did not share aspects of her own experience with them. She could not feel complacent, however, that watching her words and actions in order not to self-disclose more than what she thought would be useful to them was sufficiently effective. She was fully cognizant that much of communication is out of awareness, either in procedural or in other nonverbal forms. She could not help herself from recalling, however, reading Doolittle's (1984) memoirs about her own analysis with Freud, and how Freud pounded on the couch, declaring to Doolittle something like: "You think that just because I am an old man that I cannot be attractive to you." And she smiled to herself about being an old woman, still attractive to young men, albeit aided by the revival of patterns in each patient's past generated anew in the analysis.

But still, there was something too pleasing to her, too interesting to her about the situation, and, in her experience, too enticing. She considered various possibilities, wondering, was this a narcissistic pleasure designed to bolster a sagging self-esteem (or a sagging self?), or did she need their romantic interest in her for her own self-consolidating fantasies? Somehow it did not seem to add up.

Then the analyst had a dream. It was about her cousin Gene, whom she had not seen or thought much about for decades, but upon whom she had a crush throughout her childhood and adolescence, in actuality until she met her husband. Gene was tall, blonde, handsome, self-assured, like her patient, Bob, and when she reflected on it, she recalled that Gene, too, had become a successful lawyer. The dream itself only contained a single image of Gene, but it set her to thinking about him, about the summers they would spend together every year in the Colorado mountains, and of the relationship that had existed between them. There were four of them together every summer for 10 years: Gene; his younger sister, Ethel; the analyst's older brother, Stan; and herself. The two boys would too often during those years ignore her and go off mountain climbing together while she felt trapped at home with her much younger cousin Ethel. She had wanted nothing more than to be with the two boys, and furthermore, to want them to want to be with her, passionately to want to be with her, and ultimately, to want to be with her passionately. It came to her in a flash then. Her dreams had at last come true—a little late, a little inappropriate, but nonetheless, unconsciously irresistible.

The analyst's insight contained in her dream led not only to a change in her feelings, an increased understanding of herself, but this change in her must have been communicated to her patients as well. The analyst herself found that she was no longer especially excited to see either one of her two handsome young patients, who were no longer categorized unconsciously and automatically as her cousin and her brother. Becoming self-reflectively aware now that she had somehow collaborated with each patient's fantasies about her, and about each of them being her favorite, vying for her attention, she heard less about their competition from either of them, and they went on to deal with their own separate, unrelated problems, seeing each other less. The analyst felt much more herself in working with each of them.

It seems important to consider how this unconscious communication of the analyst's own changed feelings affected the analyses of these patients, and then how the analyst's insight directed her subsequent interactions. First, with Bob, she came to appreciate in retrospect that he had always been very attentive to her moods, to her movements, and to her every utterance. Analyst and patient had worked on this in relation to Bob's tyrannical father to whose moods he had learned to be alert in order to avoid an unpredicted explosion of his father's wrath. At the beginning of the treatment Bob would notice when his analyst moved in her chair, anticipating that she might be angry or, at the least, impatient with him. Remembering and reflecting on this aspect of the analysis, she could understand that Bob might have picked up some nonverbal and/or procedural indications of her rapt attention when he would speak of his vying with Albert for the position of favorite man, and then he might also have picked up some indication of her being less interested when he spoke of other matters. Her awareness of the possible out-of-awareness communication did seem sufficient to change Bob's self state so that he could once again focus on other matters of concern to him, and she judged it unnecessary, at least for the time, to comment upon the whole sequence of experience between them so as not to risk once again using her patient for her own needs. The analyst realized that somehow Bob had been unconsciously assimilated into an old pattern, an old self in interaction with an old other who ignored her and had not paid her sufficient attention. The analyst did not feel it necessary to address this matter with Bob because he seemed to proceed in his development not asking for or seeming to need an interpersonal-sharing experience about this episode.

It was somewhat different with Albert. Again there was a shift in Albert's self state following the presumably subtle change in his analyst's demeanor emerging out of the newly heightened self-awareness, but Albert, unlike Bob, did not turn to other matters. Instead he returned to an old theme with a new direction, a direction that led first back to his past relatedness in his family, and then to a new interest in sharing with his analyst in a more interpersonal way, a new interest in the particulars of her subjective experience: Why did the analyst seem so interested in him right from the beginning of treatment? What was there about him that appealed to her? These questions appeared, paradoxically, to be generated by the relief that he seemed to feel from her diminished attention. Her heightened attention had made him feel very uncomfortable, and in some way not known to himself. Exploration of the issue revealed that although he had enjoyed the idea of her special interest in him and the sense that he was her favorite patient, he had nevertheless felt uncomfortable with and undeserving of that status, which had repeated his early adulthood experience of guilt for having ultimately won the position of favorite son by publishing a book. He could remember more clearly what it had felt like to have been for so long the black sheep, and how his brothers might have responded in turn when his book had been published and his parents had glowed with pride in him. These reflections came in the context of Albert's analyst confirming for him that his perception of her initial interest in him was indeed accurate, that she had felt drawn to him and involved with him at the beginning in part because he had reminded her of her writer son, but that, as might be expected, that particular basis of attachment had receded as he became for her more himself, more of a person in his own right. This interpersonal exchange between them following the analyst's insight into herself and the concomitant change in their connection heightened the sense of intimacy between them, leading to and strengthening self-consolidation and consolidation of his intimate tie to the other, with the patient having stronger feelings of being himself and being recognized by the other as a person in his own right.

Turning more specifically to the issue of countertransference, it is clear that over time these patients became organized by the analyst in an old self with old other analyst–patient relational configuration. The analyst, locked unconsciously into old patterns of connection, was unable to reflect on her own feelings and locate herself accurately in time. Here the countertransference experience was corrected through insight brought about in a dream; had she not been able to self-correct in this way, we suggest that the analyses might have been disrupted, and the patients thrown off developmental course. There was a danger of the analyst unconsciously using her patients in an inverted attachment relationship, and in other ways as well that were not consistent with her keeping their needs in mind. With the self-righting insight, the relational configurations were reestablished in new–new patterns.

We want to make clear that although each of these analyses had begun and were maintained for some time in the interpersonal-sharing dimension of intimacy, once the countertransference was in place, the intimacy was no longer present. Countertransference in our framework, like transference, by definition does not allow for intimacy with the other because the other is not seen for himself or herself. When the analysis is proceeding satisfactorily, as we indicated earlier, the analyst is by definition experiencing a new–new relational configuration, and, like the patient, when in this configuration, development is ongoing, and such development continues throughout life.

Finally, the received wisdom in our field is that from the analyst's perspective, "once a patient, always a patient." We would amend this received wisdom to "once a relationship, always a relationship." That is, once the analysis is over and the contractual clinical relationship is terminated, what endures is the memory of this special relationship and the potential for a continued relationship of some kind, different but nevertheless respectful of their former connection and their ongoing needs. Moreover, termination does not seem a felicitous term or concept in our model. Some patients may continue in a much different but still clinical association with the analyst; others may feel free to return at some point in the future, and this despite other intervening forms of relatedness that may have ensued. This ongoing relatedness is part of what we include in the new–new relational configuration where the potential for interpersonal-sharing intimacy is ongoing, as well as the potential for self-transforming intimacy, and where patient and analyst continue to see and relate to one another as new persons in their own right, with needs and limits, but where the respect for the patient's developmental requirements is always kept in mind.

CHAPTER SIX

Applying Our Model to the Clinical Situation

In previous chapters we introduced important concepts from our model. These included the dimensions of intimacy (self-transforming and interpersonal sharing), the relational configurations (old–old; old–new; and new–new), and the trajectory of developmental progression (delineating the movement in the analysis from old to new, from past to present, from trauma to triumph). Taken together, these three concepts describe the positive new experience, which we postulate leads to consolidation of the self and consolidation of the intimate tie to the other. In this chapter we present detailed clinical applications of these concepts. The case vignettes are designed to illustrate how the analyst can recognize the particular dimension of intimacy emergent in the relationship and how the particular dimension guides the analyst toward optimal responsiveness. As well, the case vignettes demonstrate how to move among the different relational configurations in ways that facilitate a trajectory of developmental progression in the analytic process. Finally we illustrate what is meant by positive new experience and the variety of forms that positive new experience may take in the analytic relationship.

OLD SELF WITH OLD OTHER
AND OLD SELF WITH NEW OTHER

From Old–Old to Old–New:
The Effects of Positive New Experience

A patient entered her analyst's office in an obvious rage, refusing either to look at or to speak to him as she moved to her customary place, remaining silent for an unusual length of time. The analyst was surprised and taken aback by her mood. After a pause, he noted to her that she appeared angry, adding that her anger in the past had often been accompanied by the same marked, silent state that she was showing then. When she continued to remain silent for a few minutes, he added that also in the past, her anger had been in response to an action on his part that had hurt her. The patient responded with barely controlled anger, "You let me feel it is good to need you, but when I do, you reject me."

The analyst reflected to himself on what this might be about and remembered he had been unable to change an appointment time the day before, as she had requested. He then said, "Perhaps you felt my refusal to change an appointment time with you was rejecting." Then the patient exploded in a tirade of rage, obviously released from the protective silence in which she had entered the office, unable either to stop herself or to lower her voice. "Well, it *is* rejecting. You told me that I should let you know when something didn't feel right to me, and it didn't feel right to have to wait to see you when I really would have felt more relieved to see you earlier, before seeing my dermatologist. I wanted to see you first. You know very well how worried I was about the mole, and you said to say if I needed you. You know he could only see me at our appointment time, and I didn't want to wait until after I saw my dermatologist to see you. Then you actually said that it would be O.K. if I had to miss my hour altogether if the dermatologist couldn't see me a little later instead of at our time. How could you have been so unfeeling? You know how I worry about myself, how scared I was about that mole. How could it help me not to see you at all? I had to see you, which in itself makes me angry, and then you won't even make it easy for me. Even though you've asked me to change my hours when it suited you; how come it doesn't work in reverse? What's the point in my telling you something about what I want if you aren't going to respond? And if you think that your just knowing that I want something from you is enough, you're wrong! I know you said you wished you could be more accommodating, but I don't believe you. You didn't really try. You just said, 'No.' I think you really want to frustrate me, and you don't care if it hurts."

The analyst considered that the patient's view of him as frustrating and hurtful might be an old–old relational pattern recalling her experiences with her sadistic father, but he also considered that he may indeed have been too abrupt, too thoughtless. He at first attempted to clarify the situation, wondering whether she remembered that he had in fact offered her another time, a later hour, if she found that the dermatologist could not give her a different appointment. When the patient again became mute in response to this query, the analyst realized that his patient could not even hear him, that she was forced by her analyst's comment into the familiar self-protective strategy of angry silence. He therefore tried a different approach. He realized, in this instant that is, that his patient could not conceptualize that her analyst might have a sense of reality and of what had happened between them that was different from her own. Yet he remained unwilling to relinquish completely his own experience of their interaction. He noted quickly, without too much silence inter-vening, that perhaps his having offered the later hour nevertheless seemed to her to be as rejecting as if he had offered her no hour at all, as if he were saying something like she did not have to see him at all that day. She responded, apparently feeling heard, "Yeah! Because it wasn't what I wanted. I wanted to see you first, for you to give me an earlier time, then see the doctor at our time, and then have you call me after. I wanted to feel your concern, before, during, and after. I could care less if it didn't fit with your schedule."

Here, the analyst responded, "Well, I wish I could have done that, because that is what you felt you needed to help you through this difficult time." After a pause, the analyst, feeling that his patient's anger was subsiding, wondered aloud how it might have felt to her had he been able to be that responsive. The patient's spontaneous reply was surprising; she said, "That might have scared me. You might have seemed too worried, like there was something really for me to be scared about, or else why would you forget the others to take care of me? I guess it's impossible to be me and to get what I need, even from you." The analyst added, "That sounds to me like what you have described about being a child; your father would treat you with cruelty, but when you asked for help from your mother, she would get so anxious she couldn't be helpful. Maybe it will be different with me, that you can both ask for help and also depend on me both to want to respond and at the same time to not be so overwhelmed by your need for it." The patient was able to acknowledge, "It's conceivable, at least," and to end this clinical moment feeling less angry and more in balance.

This example presents in a very basic way what we mean by a developmental progression within the analytic process, a movement from an old–old relational configuration to a beginning old–new relational configuration through the medium of a positive new expe-rience. The patient moved, with the analyst's help, from a beginning stance in which there was a reenactment of the past in the present. First, she felt he was like her father, and she reacted with angry protracted silence followed by an uncontrolled rage in response to an other perceived as wishing to hurt; then, she imagined she would have felt like he was like her mother, helpless, anxious, and overwhelmed by her need; and finally, she moved to a beginning recognition that her analyst might be "conceivably, at least" different from both. This response on her part, a marker of the developmental progression from the old–old relational configuration to the old–new relational configuration, was facilitated by the analyst's communication of a wish to have been helpful.

To look at this clinical instance more closely, the analyst read accurately his patient's nonverbal and procedural cues, slowly bringing her to the point where she could verbally express her feelings without a sense of overwhelming shame at having to lose face, and at the same time helping her to regulate the stressful, uncontrollable rages that she had suffered in connection with her father and then with her analyst. At one point he attempted to clarify the situation by reminding her that he had indeed offered her another hour, with the goal of ascertaining to what degree there was a shared reality between them, but then added quickly that offering the later hour might have seemed to her as rejecting as if he had offered her no hour at all. In this instance the analyst moved briefly into his own subjective view of what had happened between them, before returning to his sense of her perspective on the matter. The patient's response, the "Yeah," confirmed that she knew he had offered her another time, but had felt and continued to feel that that was an inadequate response to her needs, that she had wanted to feel the analyst's concern, and that she was not interested at all in the analyst's own requirements for himself in their relationship. Although the patient thus wished for experiences that would regulate her with the other, she was not yet able to experience that self-regulation in a self-transforming other dimension of intimacy. Her immersion into a traumatic rage state kept her in an old–old relational configuration where past was all-defining and present did not exist. At this point the analyst allowed himself to express his intention to be helpful, and then, noting the patient's reduced dysphoria, felt it worthwhile to explore further how she might have felt had he responded differently by offering her a more suitable time. Her response took them both by surprise. She speculated more reflectively that he might have then seemed to her to be too concerned like her mother had been, which might have worried more than relieved her, had he acceded to her request. Her self-reflection would seem to indicate an emerging old–new relational configuration. She returned to a somewhat hopeless state in her remark that "I guess it's impossible to be me and to get what I need," but then, her addition of "even from you" indicated a beginning awareness that things should be different, that he was different from others in her life. The analyst picked up on this affect. He first made a genetic connection, and then augmented her feeling that he was different, adding that in the future she might be able to ask for help and depend on him to be able to handle it for both of them, that neither of them would be overwhelmed by her needs. This is the positive new experience that informs the dimension of intimacy present and the relational configuration that has evolved. Thus, the movement along the developmental trajectory takes place from old to new.

Finally, the foregoing example illustrates the concept of the old self with old other patient–analyst relational configuration, concerning the analyst's report of the process of patient and analyst co-constructing the narrative between them. Hence, our commentary is focused on the analyst's ongoing conception of what is happening to the patient in the exchange between them, on what is presumed to be the patient's subjective experience. It is important to note once again that the analyst has his own experience in the analytic exchange, his own set of feelings toward himself and the patient, (referred to here as the analyst–patient, as opposed to the patient–analyst, relational configuration). Other clinical examples in this chapter will more pointedly reflect the other side, or, alternatively both sides, of the mutually influencing, bidirectional relational configuration that we see as always present in the patient–analyst dyad.

From Old–New to Old–Old and Back to Old–New: When Remaining in the Old Is Traumatic

The trajectory of developmental progression is not linear, however; that is, it does not necessarily move from old–old to old–new to new–new, but may follow many patterns as determined by the patient's developmental needs. This point is illustrated in the following example of a patient who moves from an old–new relational configuration to an old–old relational configuration with her analyst.

The patient had been sexually abused when she was 13 by her maternal uncle. She had been overweight throughout elementary school, but as she entered puberty, she seemed to herself to have emerged suddenly as slim and round, with curves that she felt in retrospect had gotten her into trouble and proved to be sources of danger. Her uncle had seemed friendly and safe until she developed sexually, but then, as if in response to her pubertal changes, he, without warning, became sexually aggressive and demanding. The patient was forced under threat of physical injury to submit to his fondling her and to his involving her in experiences of mutual orgasm. She was terrified of her own sexuality and feared exposure to her mother's wrath about her behavior with her uncle. Temporary relief came when her uncle left the country unexpectedly, and as if in reaction to this regained sense of safety, she began gradually to gain weight, consciously feeling that if she were fat, she would be spared the attentions of men and she would go back to being a sexually unaware and good little girl. She found, however, that neither her fear nor her sexual desire left with the gain of weight. She struggled throughout adolescence and into college and graduate school, finding herself either inappropriately involved in sexual relationships with unreliable men or, more often, alone.

When the patient was 23, she entered into analysis with a woman analyst with complaints of intractable obesity and difficulty in relating socially. Patient and analyst formed a close and affectionate working relationship wherein the patient found herself able for the first time to tell her story, express her pain, and feel some relief in the comfort and enhanced understanding that the analysis provided. She began, only tentatively at first, to risk dieting and losing weight, but found herself helplessly stymied once she had been rewarded with pounds lost and attention gained from men. Her analyst interpreted her conflict as that she both wanted to be and feared being attractive to men, but the interpretation was useless to the patient. The analyst then went further, wondering if the patient might be feeling more afraid now to lose weight because she was already feeling attractive, reminding her that the fear was of something that had happened in the past, but that now the danger was over, and she was no longer a little girl who had to submit to her uncle. This interpretative intervention had a surprisingly strong negative effect. The patient became enraged and stormed out of the office, threatening to leave treatment forever. The analyst, confused and disturbed by her patient's upset, left a message on the patient's answering machine expressing her concern and wondering how the patient was doing. Because the relationship between them was good, the patient came back the next day, though in obvious pain. She was apologetic and confused about her own behavior. It became clear with discussion that neither analyst nor patient had quite understood the strength of the patient's terror, nor the evocative power the state of feeling attractive had for her. The analyst had assumed, mistakenly, that the patient had consciously experienced herself as already sexually desirable when, in fact, the patient did not feel that, nor could she bear even to hear of that possibility from her analyst. The analyst's words had served as a retrieval cue, recalling the uncle's numerous assaults, the sense of helplessness, the rage that her helplessness engendered, and the feeling that she must get out at all cost. It was clear to both that the direction of their work together had to be focused on how dangerous the world became when the patient saw herself as without the protective armor of excessive weight, that the problem stemming from her past abuse was not to be so simply solved.

We include this vignette to illustrate the movement of a relational configuration from an apparently solid and established old–new pattern, the patient feeling comfortable and safe in an ongoing way in the analyst's presence, but still struggling with experiences in her past, to an old–old pattern, which was familiar but which she had never before experienced in connection to her analyst, and then back to the old–new, more stable pattern that had been established and was more expectable between them once the disruption was resolved.

The analyst's phone call to her patient following the disruption indicated not just her concern and confusion, but also her sense that the patient's remaining in an old–old configuration would not be helpful or useful to their work, at least not until something of the meaning of that old–old pattern had been understood between them. The fact that this is not always the case will be addressed. But for the patient portrayed above, a positive new experience moving her out of old–old was essential to this particular patient's psychological functioning. It was deemed by her analyst to be detrimental for her to remain in a state in which the fear engendered by the flashback was overwhelming. The analyst postulated that such a state was likely to promote further self-disintegration, rather than self-integration. For the time being, at least, retrieval cues that threatened the patient's tenuously regulated state were conceptualized by the analyst as harmful to her patient, and thus to be ameliorated and contained. Presumably, as the relationship deepened further, the patient might be able to live through and put into narrative form the dysphoria connected to the old experiences of trauma, but at that time the analyst did not feel it was desirable. The rationale, based on trauma theory, is that whereas the patient's reliving in the context of safety with the person of the analyst is a helpful experience, reliving in the context of disruption constitutes an interference with the patient's developmental progression toward self-consolidation. The choice the analyst made was to regain the old self with new other constellation. In the future, in the context of a close connection, the past could be revisited, perhaps even revived, without subjecting the patient to an experience of disruptive, dangerous fragmentation.

Allowing the Patient to Remain in Old–Old

Another point can be made here. In the previous case example, the patient left the analyst's office in a rage, and the analyst opted to call her. In another instance, and with another pair, the patient might leave an analyst's office in a rage, but this analyst, with this patient, would not call, but, rather, would anticipate that his patient would reconstitute and return to the next appointment as expected. Previous experience with this patient would lead that analyst to believe the patient's fragmentation to be fleeting and manageable by the patient on her own. Or, with another patient, a call would be experienced as demeaning and patronizing. Again, we remind ourselves that the patient–analyst pair constitutes a system in which what is advantageous or necessary at one time or with one patient or between that patient and a given analyst may be quite different under different circumstances. The guideline remains a consideration of the action or reaction that might best contribute to the ongoing developmental progression, what allows the best possibility for self- and mutual regulation, and self- and mutual reflection, and what best contributes to the patient's self-consolidation and consolidation of the intimate tie to the other.

Premature Disruption of Old–Old:
The Analyst's Countertransference

Here is another example: In this case, the analyst clearly was made too uncomfortable by her patient's sense of despair to allow the patient to remain in that state for very long, especially when she was the source of his current misery, and despite the fact that there was indeed nothing that she could actually do to remove the patient's distress. The analyst understood that what was needed was to be able to stay with the patient and hear him out, but she found herself too often unable to do so. This recurrent problem came up especially each time the analyst was planning to be away from the office. In the instance to be reported here, the analyst was scheduled to attend a meeting where she was to appear on the program, but had been loathe to confront her patient with the fact that once again she would be leaving town. She kept delaying, though she had already told others in her practice. One day the patient came in waving an announcement of the upcoming program with the analyst's name on it, and said, with heavy sarcasm, "I wonder when you were planning to tell me about this one!" The analyst, caught in an all too common state of embarrassment with the patient, apologized and waited for the storm, which did come, just as she had known it would. The patient first took advantage of the analyst's obvious mistake and felt empowered to be critical and righteously demeaning, but then fell into the familiar old–old relational configuration of abandoned self in relation to a traumatically abandoning other. This was familiar enough, and after a time, the analyst did what she had often done in the past; she tried to reassure him that he could call her when he needed to, and that, in addition, she would be willing to schedule an extra appointment the following week to replace some of the time she would be gone. The patient insisted that this would not help, that the abandonment was unbearable, and that her pretending to understand and be helpful by offering to talk on the phone just made him all the angrier and all the more upset. There is nothing more upsetting, he told her, then to have an analyst who does not understand.

However, this time there was a difference; the fact that the analyst had actually gone so far as to wait to tell her patient until the patient discovered it for himself forced her to reflect on what was going on within her. The result of this self-reflection allowed the analyst to back off and to listen while the patient railed against her, offering no further avenues of reassurance. Through this process the patient remained angry and felt abandoned for the next several weeks, with the analyst becoming increasingly aware of both her own discomfort in the situation, and the necessity to bear it. It became clear that what the patient had been trying to tell her was absolutely correct: that she was unwilling to listen; that she would go to great lengths not to have to hear, because she was so eager to mollify him; and that these efforts on her part were truly disruptive, blocking the opportunity to relive in the present experiences from the past and to make the necessary genetic- and transference-based connections. Thus, with this new understanding on the analyst's part, an old–old relational configuration was, rather than being prematurely interrupted, allowed to remain in place for as long as it took for the patient to feel that his despair could truly be met and responded to by his analyst's quiet acceptance of the unbearable and inevitable pain felt by both when she disappointed him. Furthermore, the lesson the analyst learned was that it had been her own pain, rather than his, that she could not tolerate, that she had had to ameliorate by palliatives such as calls and extra sessions.

We want to make the point that we are not saying calls and extra appointments should not be made, but only that offers such as these should not come prematurely. This patient was finally permitted to revisit for as long as was needed whatever traumatic experience from the past the situation with his analyst evoked, permitted to revisit this traumatic experience in the safety that a truly available analyst provided. Previously, this safety did not exist because the analyst was unable to provide it—she herself did not feel safe in the situation. It is important to note that, in this example, an old self with old other, *analyst–patient* relational configuration was in process, a relational configuration taken from the perspective of the analyst that constitutes our definition of countertransference. The analyst, in her self-reflection, was able to get in touch with her own shame and guilt about her ambition to receive public acclaim, to put herself forward over the needs of others, an ambition that she feared was at times more important to her than her patients' well-being. Having been told forcefully as a child that it was not appropriate for girls to put themselves forward and disregard others in doing so, her personal strivings were a guilty and shameful secret hidden even from herself. This illustrates what we mean when we say that analysis is a developmental experience for analyst as well as patient.

Old–New to Old–Old: The Analyst's Personal Needs in Conflict with the Provision of Positive New Experience

There is another important concern here: Within the selfother system that constitutes the analytic situation, the analyst's needs must also be taken into consideration. To provide an example, a patient asked her analyst to call her that evening, in order to arrange a referral for her son who had become suddenly disturbed while away at college. She required that the analyst call at a particular time so that his call would not interrupt other calls that she expected from two of her friends. The analyst found himself in a bind: Having first agreed to make the call, he then remembered too late that the time his patient had requested for the phone contact, and that he had agreed to, was inconvenient. Moreover, he was aware of feelings of resentment at the patient's apparently excessive sense of entitlement. He could not help but recognize his feeling of being put down, belittled, and considered unimportant in contrast to the others in the patient's life, her friends from whom she expected phone calls, and especially in contrast to the patient herself. These feelings only came to him after the patient had left the office. He decided his best course was to leave a message for the patient informing her that, as it turned out, the time she requested did not work for him, offering to make an earlier call to her. The patient did not respond until they met as scheduled the next day at which time she vigorously berated him for breaking his promise to her. The analyst reflected to himself about what had actually motivated his decision, whether the time was really so inconvenient, or whether he had acted out of injured pride. He decided that both of his responses were valid in this case, but acknowledged to himself that his patient's needs were also important. Acting on the information he had, he concluded that his own needs required a primary place in this instance, and that his response was not based mainly on feelings of narcissistic hurt. As the patient continued her accusations, the analyst considered interpreting the patient's only partly disguised wish to devalue him, but again, based on what he knew at that moment, he opted to listen further rather than to intervene. What came out was his patient's anxiety about displeasing her friends and about being required by him to give up her friends if she was to maintain a secure connection with him. She told him that he clearly could not under-stand how important her friends were to her, and how risky it seemed to jeopardize in any way her relationships with them. Finally, he entered into a dialogue with his patient, agreeing that he had not understood the full extent of her concerns, but that nevertheless, even had he understood more, he would still have felt moved to decline her requirement to call only at that particular time so inconvenient to him. He felt more himself with this patient at this point; because he better understood his patient's motives, he no longer felt devalued by her, recognizing that her response that seemed to him excessively entitled was motivated by a self-protective strategy. What came out in further exploration was her sense that in her childhood she had always had to suppress any wishes to expand beyond her immediate family circle because the rule there was that family came first, and friends only a remote second. In this instance then, he represented the patient's demanding parents.

In this example, the patient moved from an old–new relational configuration to an old–old relational configuration at the point when her analyst's needs took priority and he did not provide the positive new experience she sought and might have benefited from. Providing this experience would have required of the analyst that he ignore important needs of his own. This, at least on the face of it, is not a countertransference response, but rather an instance where two people in an intimate relationship have conflicting needs. The analyst's responsibility in such a case is first to understand where the conflict lies between them, and to then reflect on to what extent, if any, his or her actions are motivated by a response to the patient based on the analyst's perception of the patient as a person from the analyst's past. Where the analyst, on self-reflection, does not believe this is the case, what remains is to continue to explore and to understand the inevitable tension that exists between two people whose wishes and needs may not coincide. The weight, of course, is tilted toward the patient's developmental needs, but, again, not at the expense of what the analyst feels he or she can do with comfort. Consistent with our systems view, what constitutes a legitimate need or a constraint will vary from analyst to analyst. What he or she provides toward a positive new experience for the patient will also vary from analyst to analyst, and will be in part a function of what the given analyst is able and willing to do.

ANALYSIS UNBOUND: BOUNDARIES FROM A DEVELOPMENTAL SYSTEMS SELF PSYCHOLOGY PERSPECTIVE

This last illustration introduces the issue of the analyst as well as the patient having needs and wishes that must be recognized, and raises the question of how these needs and wishes might be responded to in a well-functioning analytic relationship. There are some guidelines to follow in responding to this important clinical concern. We are addressing this concern from the perspective of the analyst because it falls to the analyst by and large to guide and preserve the analytic process, though of course such guidance and efforts at preservation are done in negotiation with the patient. One guideline is that the analyst must remain as aware as possible of his or her own self needs, including a knowledge of his or her limitations. Another guideline is to remain as aware as possible of the patient's needs as they pertain to the patient's development. It is through reflection on the ways in which these two guidelines intersect in the intersubjective-interpersonal field that the analyst is helped to determine a particular decision in any particular moment occurring in the relationship. Such a decision is traditionally referred to as a boundary decision, because it relates to what is called the analytic frame, the fairly set and established conditions under which the analysis is conducted.

In our model, we choose to maintain the term "boundary," but to emphasize the systems nature of any boundary concern, its linear and nonlinear aspects. The aspects of the boundary that are linear—that is, that are organized by cause-and-effect connections, are viewed as preset, are seen as predictable, and are more or less unvarying in nature—are in the main determined by external legal and ethical constraints imposed on the dyad. Over a period of time, these external constraints may change, but for the most part, legal and ethical codes impose fixed boundaries. Most essentially, these boundaries are predicated on the assumption that a given prohibited action is prohibited because the outcome of putting it into action will have a specific, predictable, detrimental effect. For example, ethical codes and legal codes in the mental health profession all prohibit sexual contact between patient and analyst, and they do so because it is considered certain that the outcome of such contact would be harmful to the patient and to the process.

In contrast, nonlinear boundaries are not preset, and are based neither on predictable cause-and-effect connections nor on unvarying standards, but rather on personal and interpersonal considerations, as well as on the constraints arising individually and interpersonally in the dyad. What is available or imposed changes in response to where both the patient and the analyst are developmentally. Finally, community and scientific standards as well as theoretical ideals do play a role, of course, but the role they may play depends on how flexible both analyst and patient may be in response to them. Some examples follow.

An intermittently psychotic patient suffered from profoundly disruptive negative affect states. She refused medication, but she was willing to maintain what amounted to a six to seven times per week session frequency, with either one or two weekend phone contacts sustaining her in addition to the five face-to-face sessions on weekdays. One symptom of the patient's severe fragmentation was her repeated outbursts of protracted screaming that would last for entire sessions over several weeks, alternating with periods of relative calm during which gradual progress could be ascertained by both patient and analyst. Each time the patient entered into a screaming phase, her analyst would herself become anxious and far less able to sustain an empathic and reflective state. The analyst more or less simply held herself together and endured during these phases, dreading each session; feeling inadequate, guilty, and ashamed because of this dread; and being reduced at times merely to hoping that her patient's state would shift. What troubled her most was her sense that if she could simply maintain her own good feelings toward the patient during the periods of screaming, and above all stay calm within the storm, such calm might foreclose the patient's entry into the screaming phase, or at the least help her to come out of it sooner. But feelings of tension within herself, and even rage, would become apparent to the analyst no matter what efforts she extended against such feelings, so that for the most part when the patient became fragmented to the point of screaming, both were forced simply to endure—the analyst, the patient's screaming; and the patient, her own unbearable, disrupted state.

The analyst sought supervision on this case on a number of occasions, wanting to determine first of all what she herself might do differently, and second, to what extent her own responses were countertransferential, requiring further self-analytic self-reflection, or even further analysis. Through such repeated courses of supervision, very few helpful interventions were suggested, but she was provided an opportunity to explore and reflect on her own reactions. She finally reached the awareness that although another analyst might find it within himself or herself to sustain with more equanimity these screaming periods, it was not within her own capacities to do so. Although she was able to make genetic connections to her responses to this patient, nevertheless, this inability remained an aspect of her own limitations, not changeable in herself. Further, even were such limitations in herself resolvable by another analysis, she was not willing to undertake this large project at that time. Thus a boundary arose that required that the patient be prevented from extended outbursts. The analyst told her patient that she did feel it was the patient's legitimate right to scream, and that it might well be in the patient's best interests to do so, that it might even help her to get better. Nevertheless the analyst could not work effectively with the patient when she screamed. The analyst added that someone else might be able to do so, and that she even wished she herself could, but that in fact she could not and was no longer willing or able to try. She presented the patient with a strategy she had arrived at alone, not one mutually negotiated between patient and analyst. Were the patient to scream beyond what the analyst felt she could bear, the patient would be given the option to stop screaming if she could, or leave the office, with the hope that the next day she would be feeling better. In turn, the analyst promised she would attempt to remain in contact with the patient and to understand what had promoted the patient's felt need to make herself heard with such force. The effect of this boundary imposition, although by no means a complete solution, was to help the analyst not feel so tense and so helplessly angry, which did seem to reduce the frequency and length of the patient's fragmentation states. Clearly this was not an ideal situation, as the patient no doubt felt forced, and, indeed, actually *was* forced, to comply with the analyst's limitations. Nevertheless, the boundary did make it possible for the analyst to continue the work with comfort and a sense of having regained her competence as an analyst.

This case underscores our belief that establishing boundaries must take into consideration both the patient's and the analyst's well-being. To the extent that the analyst's well-being conflicts with the patient's well-being, the patient's development may have to be compromised, at least temporarily. In an analysis unbound by tradition, then, boundaries emerge as pertinent in the dyad, boundaries that cannot be easily generalized to other times, other places, other pairs. Such issues as fee, payment arrangements, length of sessions, mutuality in experience sharing, use of touch, social contacts outside of analysis are all, ideally, addressed in each unique dyad, with the good of the patient kept paramount, but with the needs of the analyst kept in mind as well.

This is even more the case in child analysis, incidentally, where fluidity in boundaries is the rule; it is a given that a child–analyst pair will routinely arrive at rules of contact and safety that may only pertain to a single session, not to the entire analysis, much less to other analytic dyads. For example, were a child ill or deeply disturbed, he or she might be held on the analyst's lap; or, were a child in a rage, he or she might require physical restraint or containment; or, were a child particularly angry and in the habit of physically striking out at anyone around, the analyst might accept, at least temporarily, a new ability to destroy an object in the room instead; or, finally, were an adolescent discovered to be taking dangerous drugs, the analyst might with or without warning feel it was imperative to disclose this fact to the parents, realizing, of course, that the relationship would be put in serious jeopardy if not permanently disrupted.

Turning in this regard to the adult situation, were an analyst to feel in serious danger with a particular patient, he or she might choose to interrupt the treatment for self-protective purposes. For example, an analyst began work with a new patient, who, it turned out, was the daughter of a major drug lord. The analyst began to worry that her own safety might be at stake, as minor secrets from the drug ring began inadvertently to be disclosed to her. She began to worry that more serious disclosures from her patient might emerge at any time and that even if they did not emerge, a suspicion might be raised in her patient's father's mind that she, the analyst, "knows too much." When this realization dawned on her in the middle of the night, the analyst decided to terminate the treatment abruptly before the patient's father "terminated" her. She in fact discussed her fear with her patient the next morning, acknowledging that although this decision evidenced a lack of courage and fortitude in herself, she could nevertheless not continue to work effectively with the patient, risking not only her own well-being, but the well-being of her children, as well. Our point in this rather extreme example is that when the well-being of the analyst is in conflict with the well-being of the patient, the patient may well turn out to be the one who suffers.

THE NEW–NEW RELATIONAL CONFIGURATION: IS IT STILL ANALYSIS?

A patient complained to his analyst about his wife, boss, and mother. They did not listen to him, they did not understand him, and they were all in one way or another preoccupied with their self-interest. The analyst heard all of this and could not help but wonder, Could this general complaint be applied to her as well, with the patient hiding the complaint either from her or even from himself? The analyst then ventured an exploration of this possibility, on the way to interpretation. She wondered aloud, "Could any of this apply to me?" The patient's retort both surprised her and shook her conviction, leading her to think in another way. He asserted, very positively, "On the contrary! It is only here with you that I have learned what it feels like to be listened to and understood, and where my interests do seem to have significance." Were the analyst then to persist with this line of interpretation of negative transference, she would risk inducing in the patient feelings of being misunderstood, misheard, and ignored. Thus, we contend that the analyst needs to have in his or her analytic repertoire the concept of a new self with new other patient–analyst relational configuration; transference from our perspective only extends so far, and ample room is left for a novel other in the patient's life, and reflexively, a new self. Were the analyst to have no way to understand such a relational change; he or she would be more likely to retain the patient for too long in an old–old configuration, even insisting on it, and in that sense co-creating it, with no benefit accruing to the patient, to the patient's development, or to the analytic process.

This raises the question of what it means to be an analyst. An analyst knows that what is true on the surface of the patient's consciousness may only serve to disguise that which lies latent beneath, the manifest content symbolizing the underlying meaning in the patient's associations. An analyst also knows that although it is helpful to accept the patient's version of experience or truth, nevertheless there is always the potential for the analyst's being misled and being made to feel naive and foolish as a consequence. Ever since Freud abandoned his seduction hypothesis as etiological for neurosis, based on his fear that he had made a terrible error in simply believing his patients' accounts of childhood sexual abuse and sexual activity, analysts have come to err on the side of disbelieving their patients' accounts. In this way they seek to avoid repeating Freud's humiliating experience of accepting with too much gullibility their patients' memories. Concepts of unconscious fantasy, screen memory (Freud, 1899), and the family myth (Kris, 1956) have come into ascendance. Not running the risk of being naive or of being deceived by the patient has become a hallmark of the initiated, sophisticated analyst, creating a dilemma around how to listen to the patient's associations and recollections, how to stay within the patient's perspective and yet remain an analyst who attends to the hidden depths.

Another historically based dilemma lies within the analyst's justifiable appreciation for transference as a universal and powerful phenomenon. Every analyst knows that it is the transference valence that is missed by the nonanalyst, that it may well be transference that lies behind most of what the patient is ostensibly talking about, and that it is the transference and its interpretation that is the fulcrum of successful treatment. This conviction compels the analyst to look always and everywhere for transference intrusion and to interpret it consistently. The danger here lies, of course, in seeing transference everywhere, including where it is not, and in interpreting everything the patient says as constituting an unconscious reference to the patient–analyst relationship.

A third dilemma facing the analyst is the complexity inherent in all emotional states; by simply accepting what is on the surface of any emotional expression, there is a danger of missing what is also there, what is also, less consciously, felt by the patient. Here is the origin of the analyst's fear of missing the negative transference, of not interpreting aggression, or of being fooled by the patient's idealization or by any other expression of positive regard. On the other side, there is the danger of taking too literally the patient's anger, and overlooking thereby the patient's underlying, hidden love, or libidinal desire. One strategy to avoid these pitfalls is consistently to interpret the unconscious presence of a hidden affect, often the opposite one, but this in itself constitutes another pitfall, the patient feeling not listened to and misunderstood.

These three strong clinical predilections, the fear of appearing naive, the fear of missing a transference manifestation, and the fear of taking the patient's manifest expression of emotion too concretely, at face value, although understandable and clearly useful to a point, all present the potential for being themselves taken too literally by the analyst and then applied too broadly. Our point here is that these three time-honored cornerstones of psychoanalytic education, although important in and of themselves, can threaten the emergence and sustenance of the new self with new other relational configuration, thus disrupting the potential for positive new experiences.

ATTAINING AND SUSTAINING THE NEW SELF WITH NEW OTHER RELATIONAL CONFIGURATION

The Interpersonal-Sharing Dimension of Intimacy

In earlier chapters we introduced four detailed examples of new–new relational configurations in ongoing analytic work. The first appeared in Chapter 1 and concerned the woman traumatized by her psychotic mother who had attempted to smother her with a pillow. If you remember, this patient had felt immediately in the analysis and for the first time in her life a positive new experience of safety and security, a new self with new other patient–analyst relational configuration that was ongoing throughout the treatment. The next three illustrations of the new–new relational configurations appeared in Chapter 3, concerning dimensions of intimacy, and included discussion of how expressions of love can be dealt with as instances of the appearance of the self with new other relational configuration in the analytic relationship.

What follows now is a case illustration in which the analyst deliberately decided to share an experience of his own that matched an experience of his patient's, thereby initiating an interpersonal-sharing dimension of intimacy, and introducing into the dyad a new self with new other relational configuration. Here the analyst was risking the creation of an impasse, which might have resulted from an intemperate intrusion into the patient's private world of experience.

A married woman in her third year of analysis, whose sense of her analyst was greatly influenced by a wishful idealization of him as a strong and protective paternal figure, returned from a vacation during which she and her husband had visited the Freud Museum. She graciously presented her analyst with a small gift from the museum and described some reactions to the experience. Being herself a therapist, she had some expectation of being treated to a warm and cordial reception at the museum, and was disappointed at what she perceived as an atmosphere of coldness and an air of distance in the personnel. The analyst deeply resonated with her response. He was tempted to share his own experience with visiting the Freud site in Hampstead some years before, but hesitated to do so, knowing that to go down that road would require considerable self-disclosure with unpredictable outcome. He somehow felt nevertheless that in the end it would be beneficial to the patient as well as enjoyable to himself to talk over with her his similar view of the emotional tone generated in the Freud Museum. He knew that his patient idealized him; but he knew also that what was less accessible to her was a growing sense of herself as his equal, with a shared humanity between them. His affective resonance, his wish to share his story with her, and some idea of developmental progression taking place in her all added up to revealing the following story about himself.

As President of the Anna Freud Foundation in 1980, he and his wife were privileged guests of Anna Freud herself. Before taking them personally to the Hampstead Clinic Nursery School (now referred to as the Anna Freud Centre), where the three would spend the morning visiting with the children, Anna Freud asked if they would like to visit her father's study. He and his wife were then led into what seemed to the analyst to be a pharaoh's tomb. Preserved intact was Sigmund

Freud's consultation room, complete with its pyramid of pillows on the couch, the incredible cascade of Persian rug; the behind-the-couch chair; all the pictures, statues, paraphernalia, and psychoanalytic volumes; and the desk and cracked leather desk chair itself, with an open book and the papers and pen that Freud had been working with at the time of his death. The analyst felt very somber both in Anna Freud's presence and in the presence of this room, but his wife, who was less easily awed by the situation, turned humorously to her husband and said, "Why don't you sit down at the desk; maybe it will rub off and help you write like Freud." Before he could respond in kind, Anna Freud intervened abruptly, in some apparent alarm, and said, with abrasiveness, "I think not!" The matter was summarily dropped. But her coldness, her lack of humor in relation to anything close to her father, her failure to respond with even a modicum of empathy and responsive understanding, had lingered with the analyst to that time, resonating with his patient's story. And it was this strong reawakened impression that proved irresistible to him as he recounted the experience.

The patient responded by expressing her feeling of being nonplused at this uncharacteristic behavior on the part of her analyst, saying, "I can't believe you're telling me this story, but I love it." She then went on in a way that slightly worried her analyst, saying, "Imagine! You actually knew this person who was so close to Freud!" The analyst was surprised by his patient's awe. Moreover, he was disturbed because, having heard this response, he feared in retrospect that his disclosure had been motivated by an unconscious, grandiose, narcissistic wish to display his august connections, and because his patient was anyway too prone to idealization. But, as it turned out, she perceived his response in a much more complex, in-depth way than he could have anticipated, understanding him better than he could have imagined she would. She experienced the analyst's behavior as his wish to establish equality between them, in effect to diminish her idealization of him and to introduce a more intersubjective engagement with him, and she was grateful for this expression on his part. Again, the patient's response to her analyst's unspoken set of motives reflects the bidirectionality inherent in the dyad; just as he was able to predict her wish for greater shared intimacy, so she was able to comprehend and value his own wishes for shared interpersonal intimacy.

The complexity of the patient's response emerged in a dream told to her analyst the following day. She reported the dream as follows: "I have been thinking about this dream all day. It opened in a shabby, large penthouse in Vienna. I know this is a reference to Freud. I was sitting on a hard-backed chair. You were behind me, not sitting but kneeling. Our heads were on the same level. I had my back to you. I put my hand up and you clasped it and said, 'Just for today, we won't have an analytic relationship; we are going to be like friends.' It wasn't sexual. You said, 'I think we should go to a play together.' " The patient then interjected, "I think the dream and this comment has to do with playing together, having fun." She then went on with the dream: "I went down some stairs, and instead of joining you at the play, I found myself situated in a cubby or alcove with a little peephole watching you watching the play." The patient's further associations had to do with watching the analyst watch the play. She said, "I see you seeing things *I* want to see." This led her to describe two films she had seen in which someone is looking at two people making love, with the person looking on becoming aroused by the sight. The patient reconsidered the comment she had made earlier as she began to recount her dream that "it wasn't sexual." She went on to talk of *Alice in Wonderland*, in her association to the staircase in the dream and the small cubbyhole, and said, "Lewis Carroll was a child molester."

As the patient continued in this same vein, the analyst became slightly anxious again, thinking once more that perhaps he should not have told his vignette; he worried that his patient had organized the analyst's sharing his story as a harmful seduction of her, seeing him as a child molester who exposes her to a primal scene. He then intervened, asking his patient, "Might there be any connection in this dream to the story I told you about my wife and me and Anna Freud?" The patient responded with alacrity, "I can't believe you told me that story. I really liked it that you told me; it's just awesome, just one person removed from Freud! You and Anna Freud!" The analyst added, "And my wife." "Maybe," she responded. The analyst elaborated at this point, "A peek at something that went on between me and my wife." She answered, "Yeah, and it really surprised me. I loved that story. I did. You rarely tell me anything about yourself."

The primal scene stimulation taken from the story and reflected in the patient's dream seemed quite apparent. The idea that the analyst could have been molesting her by this stimulation was also apparent. What might have been less apparent is the patient's experience of the analyst's having come down to her level (the analyst kneeling next to her in the dream), to greet her as an equal, to let her into his life, and to share as two friends. As the analysis has progressed subsequently, it is the latter effect that has emerged as the more powerful theme, and this effect does seem to be salutary for the patient, and for the process as well. In our terms, it becomes positive new experience. Hence, with all the obvious concerns about stimulating her anxiety with an inappropriate revelation that appears to be harmfully seductive, overall, the patient took in the experience as some indication of the analyst's good-will toward her, respect for her, wish to be close to her, and wish to confide his own experience. The more brittle aspects of her idealization of the analyst faded, to be replaced by a more solid and more authentic respect for the analyst, for herself in connection to him, but also for herself alone, the experience seeming to initiate, or at least to mark, an increase in self-consolidation that was palpable and lasting.

We see this vignette as exemplifying a movement toward a new–new relational configuration, with an overlap of old–new patterns—the woman who could now talk (and dream) safely about herself as the fearful child, but who nevertheless could view her analyst as one with whom she could reflect openly about these old, newly revived anxieties. However, it was the new–new relational pattern and the interpersonal-sharing dimension of intimacy that largely predominated, with both patient and analyst taking pleasure for a time in their mutually resonating experience. We want to make the point that it is the entirety of the experience that constitutes what is positive and new in it: the capacity to tolerate the embarrassment in associating to the difficult sexual material, the capacity to reflect on and play with her own fantasies of analyst as seducer, her strong belief in her analyst as caretaker, the ease and facility in relaying and then questioning her clear idealization of him, and the more recently acquired capacity to achieve an equality in interpersonal sharing. Like any other relational configuration in analysis, the pattern fluctuates, but new–new, once attained, remains as a permanent acquisition, a potential that is then available to the pair.

To elaborate further on this vignette, it seems important to consider and explore why the analyst chose not to focus more than he did on the relatively unconscious sexual meanings and the hints at child molestation that were elicited in the patient's associations to the entire experience. Earlier we pointed to three fears that analysts carry with them in their work with patients: the fear of appearing naive, the fear of missing a transference manifestation, and the fear of taking the patient's expressions of emotion too concretely and too narrowly. These fears are important and helpful in carrying out the fullest and most complete exploration of the patient's experience with the analyst. However, from our perspective, these same fears may create in the analyst a mistrust in the ease of an ongoing positive new experience and lead to the analyst's iatrogenic maintenance of the patient in an old self with old other relational configuration. In this example, the patient's sexuality and fears of molestation did surface, and they were discussed freely and openly, so that she could associate to earlier figures of fear in her life, like Lewis Carroll, whose stories frightened her when she was a child. But these thoughts, feelings, and associative connections were revealed in the context of a newly emerging playful and safe relatedness with the analyst as a person in his own right, and it was this aspect that the analyst felt was most salient, most conducive to developmental progression. And so it was this aspect that became the more privileged for the analyst in our example, consistent with our framework in which returning a patient to an old–old constellation for its own sake is not conceptualized as enhancing development.

The Self-Transforming Dimension of Intimacy

In the following vignette there is also an emergent new–new relational configuration, but here it is the self-transforming dimension of intimacy that pertains, with only hints of interpersonal-sharing intimacy arising within the context of an impasse in the analysis. That is, a new–new configuration only became recognizable as a pattern through the experience of disruption in the dyad, with totally unexpected consequences that ensued from a spontaneous expression of the analyst's feelings, the totality creating a positive new experience.

The patient, a married woman with two children, had been in analysis for approximately 2 years, an analysis punctuated with frequent disruption and efforts at repair. Shortly before the patient was to go away on a 2-week family vacation, she heard that the youngest of her two children, a boy in sixth grade, had not been accepted by any of the secondary schools to which he had applied. The patient was devastated. All of her son's friends had been accepted to at least one school, and the family had not even considered his going to public school as an option. She called her analyst in an agitated state, something she had done only once before, and when she came into session the next day, one day before the family was scheduled to leave, she reviewed with her analyst her despair. She said that she was attempting to reach by phone the headmaster of the school they had felt he was surely going to be admitted to, the school where her older child was already enrolled in the seventh grade. She said also that she had decided not to tell her younger son about the rejections until after their vacation was over, allowing him to enjoy the trip and also allowing a period of time during which her efforts with the headmaster might bear fruit. The patient was clearly attempting to self-regulate, to modulate her distress with hopes that all would turn out well. Her analyst, however, was out of step with her patient. She was feeling some moderate anxiety of her own for the child's predicament, having worried since the day before, when she had gotten the phone call, that this would be a very difficult situation for the family, and more specifically for her patient, were it not somehow remedied. She broke into the patient's efforts to calm herself, instead of retaining her more customary stance with this patient of trying to remain with the patient's experience, by asking a question consciously intended to pacify her patient and to share with her patient the benefits of her own expertise about educational institutions in the community. In retrospect, however, this out-of-the-ordinary intervention had been unconsciously designed to reassure the analyst herself. The analyst asked her patient, "Have you thought of the public school in your neighborhood, which I know to be a good one?" During the session the patient complied with her analyst's unconscious need for reassurance, responding to the question with her own thoughts on the matter, but 2 hours later, as the family was preparing to depart from the city, she called in a rage, leaving a message on the analyst's voice mail. She shouted into the phone, "How could you do this to me? You know how upset I am about this situation, and how I was trying to cope in my own style. Maybe you don't like my style, but that is my business. Don't call me back! I don't want to hear from you. I'll see you when I get back."

The analyst spent the 2 weeks her patient was away feeling guilty, feeling responsible for the misattunement to her patient's needs, and attempting to understand her own actions. Through self-reflection, she understood that she must have been more anxious than she had realized, and she had imposed on the patient her own way of dealing with such anxiety, not to suppress it, as her patient tended to do, but to address it directly, looking immediately at the worst-case scenario, and attempting to solve the problem for the patient in the way she would have solved such a problem for herself. The analyst comforted herself with a sense that the error she had made was really not so grave, and that perhaps by the time the patient had returned she, too, would have put the unfortunate remark into perspective. In the meantime, the analyst had figured out rather belatedly, during the patient's absence, when she herself was going to go on vacation and was in the process of giving these dates to her other patients. She intended to tell this patient, too, of her vacation plans on the day the patient returned from vacation, inasmuch as she was already unusually late in informing her.

On the Monday the patient was due back, the analyst had, as was customary for her, left her appointment book open next to her, with the impending vacation dates noted, as a reminder to herself to relay this information. But contrary to her analyst's hopes, the patient came back in the same rage that had pervaded her phone message 2 weeks before. She ranted the entire hour, saying that she felt that what her analyst had intended by her remark about public school was to depress her further in an effort to keep her dependent and needy, that the analyst obviously required for her own well-being patients who were desperate and beseechingly subservient. The analyst listened, feeling dismayed but consciously resigned to the further work it would take to repair this breach, and she concluded that this was not the day after all to tell the patient about her upcoming vacation. She therefore automatically, and without conscious awareness, closed her appointment book and prepared to listen some more. But the patient became suddenly overcome with fear, broke into tears, and began to plead with her analyst not to give up on her. After some momentary confusion, the analyst realized that she had inadvertently shut her appointment book, that this closing of the book was experienced by the patient as "closing the book" on her, and that the patient was reacting accordingly. The analyst became aware further that her automatic action had been perceived by the patient correctly, that without knowing it, she did feel like closing the book on her patient, but this perception dawned on her only slowly during that day. In the meantime, the hour ended, with the patient to return the next day.

On the following day, the patient repeated her accusations at the same time that she expressed a helpless need for her analyst and, as she herself noted, an irrational fear that her analyst would get rid of her. She connected this fear of being discarded by the analyst with events in her life with her parents. The connection did allay her anxiety somewhat, but she did not desist from vehemently accusing the analyst of attempting to keep her helpless and afraid by the comment she had made prior to vacation. Again she expressed loudly and insistently her anger and her certainty that she was right, that the analyst was deliberately keeping her helpless and afraid. Finally, the analyst could no longer restrain herself. She asserted self-protectively that she had not intended to distress her, but instead, was attempting to treat her as she would have treated herself were it her own child who was about to be so wounded by rejection. Finally, she told the patient with unexpected passion that she did not mind agreeing that she had made an error, that what she had said was indeed poorly responsive to the patient's needs, that she had forgotten for the moment her patient's ways of self-soothing and had thoughtlessly imposed on her her own ways, which indeed had turned out to be most unhelpful, and that, finally, she might have been motivated to reassure herself rather than her patient. All of this she was willing to accede to, but she resented being told what her motives had been without the patient's ever inquiring about what the analyst had experienced, and without the patient ever questioning the correctness of her own conclusions. This all was said with some feeling, and with the feeling mounting as the analyst moved toward the end of her declaration. The patient was amazed. She was totally surprised by her analyst's response; felt, paradoxically, greatly relieved by it; and expressed her delight that her analyst had survived her attack rather than succumbed to it as she herself would have done, and *had* done in relation to her father so many times in her life. It seemed the impasse was miraculously and unpredictably over.

What then followed was the patient's report, several weeks later, of an exchange she had with her own child. The patient had forgotten that her youngest son had asked her to reserve a place for him in a weekend camp, and by the time she had remembered, all the places were gone. Her son was furious. He ranted at her, outraged that she had forgotten and that now he would have to miss out. He went on to accuse her of doing this to hurt him, telling his mother that it was only because it was he, not his older brother, who had made the request, that she never would have made such a mistake with his brother, that she loved his brother more, hated him, and wanted to punish him. All of the patient's efforts to apologize for her mistake and to reassure her youngest son that she did not hate him but loved him every bit as much as she loved his brother were not helpful; he continued to express anger and to make accusations. She allowed the outburst to go on and continued in her efforts to placate her child until her own patience wore out. Then she responded with strong feeling that she did not mind his accusing her of making an error; she freely admitted that she had done so and felt very sorry for it, but that she deeply resented his attributing to her motives that she did not have. She had not appreciated the parallel process between the experience with her analyst and the experience with her son until she was in the middle of it with him, but in later laughing with her analyst as she recounted the story, the patient insisted that she had learned a great deal from the analyst's authentic outburst. It had taught her how to deal with her own and her son's anger, and how to explore the multiple meanings inherent in any strong emotional response. In particular, she learned that she did not have either to be overwhelmed or to overwhelm the other in a given explosive exchange. She learned as well that by understanding her own and the other's motives and subjective experience in an argument, that affect itself could be mastered, becoming a part of a successful self-and-other mutually regulated emotional interchange. Finally, she learned that through such understanding, she could actually protect herself from the self-shattering aspects of vituperative outbursts in the dyad. Indeed, in the several years that have passed since this event, the experience stands out in the patient's mind as a key meliorative interaction.

In any case, from our perspective, this clinical example serves as an instance of an incipient new–new relational pattern arising in the self-transforming dimension of intimacy, replacing an old–old relational configuration. That is, the self-revelation was not experienced by the patient as an instance in which she got to know her analyst better from the analyst's subjective perspective; rather the use to which this self-revelation was put was to transform the patient's self by providing a new model for handling complex, intense emotional experience. It is for this reason, the use to which the intimate connection was put, that we term it an instance of a self-transforming rather than an interpersonal-sharing dimension of relatedness. In terms of the relational configuration, the patient moved from a reversal of a traumatic childhood experience of herself in interaction with her father wherein she had to succumb to his forceful, tyrannical outbursts of rage, to an experience of an other who, exposed to such rageful attack, responded by taking responsibility for those parts of the accusation that rang true to her, while at the same time protecting herself from attributions that rang false. This then became for the patient an other that could be used for identification and for affect recognition, differentiation, and delineation.

We should also make the point here that, in this context, the analyst determined which of the attributions made against her by the patient resonated with her own self-experience, and then, having determined for herself what seemed genuine, made that distinction for the patient. That is, she said, in effect, "Yes, you are right; I was in error; I was motivated to make myself feel better as well as to make you feel better; but I was *not* motivated, as you insist, by my need to keep you depressed and submerged for my own self-affirming purposes." Here is an instance wherein the analyst presented herself as herself, not automatically restricting herself to the patient's perspective. In this instance, then, the analyst saw herself as an arbiter of her own reality. Two points are thus important here: First, in our framework, the analyst was free to offer another, alternative perspective to the patient when such a perspective was thought to be in the patient's best interests; and, second, the analyst could assume that her perspective on herself and her motives was at least as accurate a reflection on her feelings as that offered by the patient. Neither had privileged access to reality in general, then, but we do make the assumption that both patient and analyst had the best and most accurate access to her own inner world.

Thus, the analyst provided for the patient an example of how to stand up for herself in the face of another's differing perspective, all the while remaining open to the patient's reflections about her. By so putting forward her own motives, the analyst helped the patient to realize that the motive counted, that the intention organizing the analyst's remarks was well meant. That is, to reverse a familiar aphorism, often "the road to *health* is paved with good intentions."

In conclusion, this example illustrates the often serendipitous nature of positive new experience, emerging as it does in a nonlinear fashion; the analyst did not predict, nor could she, the effects of her interventions. In the model we are proposing here, all we can do as analysts is to track as closely as possible the ongoing process and to respond when we can in ways that are designed to promote the patient's development. This same unpredictable, serendipitous achievement of a new–new relational pattern, but here with hints of an emergent interpersonal-sharing dimension of intimacy, is described below.

Gift Giving and the Positive New Experience

An analyst greeted her patient in the waiting room and was struck by the beauty of the patient's jacket lying on the chair next to where the patient was sitting. The analyst spontaneously remarked about it, commenting on the silkiness and lushness of color, and they entered the office together talking of other things. At the end of the session, which was filled with the patient's emotion concerning her ongoing relationship with her inadequately responsive mother who was currently visiting, the patient and analyst got up together. The patient lifted her jacket from the couch and quite suddenly extended her arm and said, "Here. You admire this, and I want you to have it." The analyst, nonplused, completely taken off guard, and striving to remain an analyst with an appropriate degree of restraint and self-containment, after first spontaneously reaching out to take it from the patient's hand, and noting, without wanting to, the pure pleasure of its luxurious silken feel, again just as spontaneously returned it to her patient, saying, "I simply can't just take your jacket; let's talk about it tomorrow." That night, in recalling the experience, the analyst remained unsettled, and so resolved to wait and see what would happen next.

The following day the patient returned furious, ready and fully energized to explore the encounter with her analyst. She jumped right in: "How can you be so stupid and unfeeling? You of all people know how hard it is for me to feel I have anything of worth to offer. You know how hard it is for me to take a chance and do something risky and experimental. You know how hard it is for me to assert myself at all. And yet you humiliate me by rebuffing my offer of something that belongs to me and that you like. I can only think it is because it is *mine* that it is distasteful to you, and I feel ashamed, and angry with you that you caused me to feel this way." At this point the analyst felt remorseful, confused, disturbed, and humiliated. Now she was truly uncertain as to what to do, and uncertain also as to what she should have done the day before. She responded by telling her patient that the patient's offer had been made only, after all, in response to her own expression of admiration for it, that it was not something the patient would otherwise have intended to give her, that it was not as if it were a gift she had brought in with the full expectation of presenting it. She also told the patient that she regretted how she had handled the situation up until then, that certainly she had no intention of squelching the patient's experimental mood, and that in fact the analyst's response had been based on her own awkwardness, first taking and then returning the jacket, and her own sense of being thrown off balance. With these statements the analyst intended to support the patient's new and tentative effort to assert herself, and the analyst's remarks did seem to repair the moderate impasse. This was borne out the next day when the patient, exhibiting a new resourcefulness and a fine sense of irony, ceremoniously presented her analyst with the jacket in an elaborately gift-wrapped box. The analyst this time acted with more grace, both to the gift and to the joyful and humorous spirit with which it was offered. She found in herself also a joy of her own, based on a sense of beginning intimacy and closeness with the patient. Before this incident, the relational configuration had been, primarily, in the form of an old–new pattern and the intimacy between patient and analyst that of a self-transforming connection, but around this incident we might postulate that a new–new pattern and an alteration in the intimacy connection into a interpersonal-sharing dimension was in the process of formation. Interestingly, it was the patient who took the lead and seemed to dare more, with the analyst struggling to catch up with the patient's forward-moving development and still remain an analyst whose patient's needs sustained a central place in their relationship.

It is interesting to reflect on this rather unusual experience in an analytic relationship. Evident in these interventions is the positive direction co-created by patient and analyst together. We want to remind the reader, however, that the decision taken by the analyst in this example was based on a sense of where that patient and analyst were in the relationship already established between them. In this case, the analyst did not believe that a further experience of shame and humiliation, an old–old relational configuration, would, through its further exploration, benefit the patient. As the patient herself had contended, they had explored long enough how difficult it was for her to feel that she had anything at all to offer, and how hard it was for her to risk doing something different in a relationship. Thus the analyst's ultimate decision to accept the gift was based on her sense of an emerging new–new relational configuration. In fact, given that context, we can consider in retrospect that the analyst might have simply accepted the gift, however provisionally, at the patient's first offering, with the proviso, either spoken or unspoken, that that experience of gift giving and gift receiving would require further discussion, and, perhaps, lead ultimately to a different conclusion. We wonder, that is, in retrospect, whether the latter alternative might have been better in the sense of being more seamlessly helpful to the patient, in place of the actual interchange, which had, after all, resulted in an impasse, however brief and however easily resolved. Perhaps handling the matter of spontaneous gift giving in this way was no different than handling a spontaneous question by responding with an immediate answer, also to be followed by further inquiry. We take the position that gratifying desire does not extinguish ambivalent feelings or prevent the exploration of their meaning; rather, we believe that conditions of safety and intimacy in the new–new relational configuration facilitate the patient's curiosity, exploration, self-awareness, and self-reflection, all of which features characterize a positive new experience.

Twinship Experience in the Self with Self-Transforming Other Dimension of Relatedness

The next example concerns a different self-transforming dimension of intimacy wherein analyst and patient are perceived by the patient as just alike, that is, a twinship, alter ego experience (Kohut, 1984) that serves to strengthen and sustain the patient's self and sense of basic, shared humanity.

The patient, a 35-year-old single teacher, entered treatment for help with a lifelong problem with anorexia. The patient's weight had always been just above a dangerous level. She had made several attempts at getting help, including trying biofeedback, entering therapy several times, and being hospitalized twice, once in early adolescence and once in her early 20s. Although the patient had managed thus far to remain alive, she had nevertheless suffered numerous bouts of illness and anemia reflective of inadequate nutrition, as well as a lifelong struggle with dysphoria punctuated by periods of elation while dieting. As the analyst listened to her new patient's history, she was particularly struck by the patient's sense of aloneness, as well as the patient's feeling that for her, eating would never feel good; all of her treatment, including her therapy, and her experiences with biofeedback, had been of no help in effecting a sense of pleasure and mastery. Although she had complied from time to time with the advice provided and had attempted to establish a comfortable relationship with her several therapists, she had in truth remained unhappy, feeling completely alone with her problem. She doubted that anything could be done for her in this new relationship, either.

What began to develop in this treatment that distinguished it from the patient's previous experiences was that she felt understood in a new way, a way impossible to articulate at first, but that over time took the form of a sense that her analyst somehow comprehended her struggles, reducing the feeling of being isolated from others. The patient then formed the conviction, based on her sense of being understood and known, that she and her analyst were just alike. On her side, the analyst's strong impression about her patient and her patient's experience, particularly the sense of being alone with a problem that disrupted her state of well-being on a continual basis, led the analyst first to focus on the patient's day-to-day feelings about eating, and then, in response to the patient's persistent questions, to offer to her patient her own personal struggles with this same problem. The patient had correctly assessed that her analyst's capacity to appreciate so intimately the patient's problem stemmed from the analyst's own difficulties with weight regulation, difficulties that she had already mastered, partly through her own personal analysis. This belief that the analyst was just like her facilitated the patient's ability to connect and to feel better. For example, the analyst, in response to the patient's queries, shared her own past suffering with eating, how it was to feel stuffed, how it was to feel starved, and how it was to be elated from starvation, exercise, and progressive weight loss. By sharing and matching such feelings, by disclosing her capacity to be empathic with her patient, the analyst helped the patient become empathic with herself, aware of her own self states and the denial that had been involved in maintaining a fiction about what felt good. Above all, the patient no longer felt alone; she felt instead, and for the first time, that she was with another who had suffered from and mastered similar experience. For the first time she felt herself to be a human being in connection to another human being just like herself. Through this new perception, the patient then came to understand on the deepest level how she was hurting herself with this behavior. In particular, her failure to starve herself effectively yielded a body that, no matter how thin it got, was not like her ideal image of herself, separating her from herself, and leading to feelings of self- and other alienation. Because the ideal could never be achieved, she could never meet the minimum requirement she had imposed on herself for membership in the human race, generating the inevitable sense of isolation and aloneness.

The connection between analyst and patient continued to evolve, with increased sharing. The patient would ask, "What was it like for you?" and the analyst would respond, helping the patient to know the analyst. Then the patient came to ask, "Is this what it was like for you?" indicating an increasing sense of "you are just like me." Through this process, a self- and mutual-regulatory experience of great value to the patient was initiated. The extent to which this process created a twinship, interpersonal-sharing intimacy, genuine and authentic, was indicated one day, when the patient, looking at her own carefully and precisely manicured nails, and then looking over at her analyst's more ragged, ill-kempt ones, commented with all sincerity, "Even our nails are just alike." Upon inquiry, the patient's meaning turned out to be that her own nails had been ill-kempt once and that the analyst's nails, with a little care, could be just like her own. By saying this, the patient was reflecting on the fact that she had now gained weight and was feeling better, just as her analyst felt better, and that she, in turn, could help her analyst to achieve what the patient had already achieved for herself.

We include this example to illustrate the use of circumscribed aspects of interpersonal sharing, which serve in this case to consolidate the patient's sense of self and tie to the analyst by means of a self-transforming intimacy and not an interpersonal-sharing intimacy. We are attempting to communicate, then, how selective interpersonal sharing can heighten the self-transforming dimension of intimacy, with the latter dimension still being ascendant in the connection between patient and analyst.

"Medical Rounds"

As a final example of a new–new relational configuration in a self-transforming dimension of intimacy, we will provide an illustration of work with a patient who said something like "I feel much better while I am here, and for a little while after, but it just doesn't last." It is often facilitating for such patients to be allowed some contact with the analyst in the intervening intervals that are so difficult for the patient. With some patients, just hearing the analyst's voice on the message machine is sufficient to sustain a meliorative contact; with other patients, a short, perhaps 2-minute interchange on the telephone carries the desired effect. And for still others, from time to time a more extended supplement to the analytic hours proves to be necessary. From our perspective, such responsiveness is an essential part of the analytic experience for this group. Although this may be no news to many contemporary analysts, the responsiveness itself is often done surreptitiously, shamefully, with the analyst feeling a sense of failure, that his or her work as an analyst is less effective than it should be, and that by such contingencies, the analytic frame is seriously strained or even fractured. From a different perspective, there is a fear that a malignant regression will ensue.

Our own stance is one in which, first of all, attuned responsiveness is the primary consideration. In fact, we believe that such attunement, rather than fostering malignant regression, protects against it through

consolidating the attachment tie in the secure base, leading to consolidating the patient's self. The important consideration is that the
response be helpful, be addressed to the patient's needs as assessed by
the pair, and above all, be no more than what either patient or analyst
can tolerate, reflecting again the concept addressed earlier of analysis
unbound. Our model uses neither the frame of classical analysis,
observing abstinence, neutrality, and (mainly) interpretive insight
provision; nor, alternatively, the frame of relational analysis, wherein
a resolution of this difficulty lies in further understanding and exploration within the conventional analytic setting, with the analyst
believing that if the patient cannot hold onto him or her in his or her
absence it is because not enough has been understood. We hold, in
addition, for these patients, that more than understanding and/or
analytic contact restricted to the hour are required for the patient to
remain held and to feel attached. This goes along with our view that
positive new experience is essential and can be provided, that suffering
in itself is not valuable and can be ameliorated; it is our belief that
the potential for analytic understanding, effectiveness, and success is
increased thereby.

With apologies for invoking the medical model here, and exclud-
ing all of the drawbacks of this model, we will borrow the nonpejora-
tive concept of "medical rounds" (without the extra financial charge
involved) for relatively brief contact, with the benefits of keeping in
touch with the patient's ongoing condition. There are many reasons
why patients cannot live up to the idealized model of the so-called
"analyzable" patient, a concept that, incidentally, we do not share.
First, what is required for the trajectory of developmental progression
is the ultimate attainment of experiences within a new–new relational
configuration, but such new organizations of experience are tenuous
and fragile, taking considerable time to become solid, dependable,
reliable, ongoing, and constitutive of continuous or consistently re-
trievable aspects of the new self and new self with new other (Kohut's
[1977] delicate tendrils of new structure). Second, the surround may
not provide supportive resources for the patient and may even create
stressors that serve as retrieval cues of old self states or patterns of
organization. The point we want to emphasize is that with any patient,
the new–new relational configuration must evolve in its own time.
Until then, supplemental experiences may be required, supplements
consistent with what the analyst feels capable of tolerating. An analyst
who, out of theoretical conviction, is reluctant to provide such supplements to the regularly attended analytic sessions may unknowingly

foster the very fear and self-fragmentation that constitute the feared malignant regression the analyst wishes to avoid and that serve to undermine the progress of the analysis. Such an analyst does not keep in mind the trajectory of developmental progression, which we view as central to analytic process and constitutive of analytic progress.

≫ CHAPTER SEVEN

The Clinical Situation across the Lifespan: Infancy and Childhood

In this chapter and the next we apply our approach to clinical work with infants, children, and adolescents. In one sense, however, it is artificial to distinguish sharply a therapeutic approach on the basis of age or stage of life. From our perspective, the entire lifespan is best understood through a systems model where what is conceptualized as a foreground developmental or clinical issue at one particular age remains significant but in the background at another age. Hence, many developmental clinical issues remain important throughout life, no matter what the age. For example, the young child largely uses play to communicate, but an adult, too, may turn to play on occasion to invoke salient issues that cannot be easily or successfully put into words. Thus play remains a background option at every age (M. Shane, 1968; Winnicott, 1971). To supply another example, the infant obviously requires the presence of a caregiver both in development and in the therapeutic situation, but the older child, adolescent, or even adult also benefits from the presence of a caregiving other for developmental progression. From our perspective, although what is therapeutically salient and useful does change in emphasis as the individual grows and develops, the clinician must remain open, flexible, and alert to the multipotentiality inherent in development, within and outside the clinical situation.

PSYCHOANALYTIC TREATMENT
IN THE INFANT–FAMILY SYSTEM

We will begin with a view of psychoanalytic therapeutic interventions in infancy. Such psychoanalytic interventions can occur in a brief treatment situation, or they can occur in the context of a more lengthy process. Short-term interventions can be helpful therapeutic approaches when a problem arises in the mother–infant pair, addressed effectively within several brief treatment modalities. Bertram Cramer (1992), for example, describes a convincing model for short-term work. Cramer's model is successful when the mother develops an immediate, positive, idealizing relationship to the therapist and the mother's interactions with her infant can be readily traced back to old patterns in which the infant becomes experienced by the mother as either her traumatized self from childhood or, alternatively, her traumatizing other from childhood. In such situations, the analyst is able rapidly to interpret the connection to the past, allowing the mother to perceive the baby as an individual in his or her own right and not as a revenant from earlier times. Development can then ensue. Cramer's model is not successful, however, in situations when the mother quickly develops a negative relationship with the analyst, a transference pattern in which the analyst is perceived as a traumatic other from the mother's past. In these situations, Cramer says, long-term, intensive therapy is required.

Cramer's approach stands in contrast to another well-recognized and successful therapeutic model in which the analyst concentrates exclusively in a focused manner on whatever strengths are observable in mother–infant interactions in the dyad, and in which interpretative intervention is not used at all. The mother's positive and successful parenting capacities and her individual strengths are recognized and affirmed, and improvement in the mother–infant pair results from self-esteem enhancement and reinforcement of the mother's salient gestures. This model has been put forward by Susan McDonough (1993) and incorporated into the intervention models of such innovators as Daniel Stern (1995) and Alice Wright (1996).

The approach we exemplify here is a psychoanalytic approach that integrates Cramer's (1992) and McDonough's (1993) models, but utilizes as well our concepts of relational configurations, dimensions of intimacy, and positive new experience, as described in earlier chapters. In addition, our approach emphasizes procedural experience and memory along with declarative experience and memory, as, especially in infancy and early childhood but also with patients of any age, memory organized procedurally—in nonverbal, action, and emotional patterns—is important to consider, and may at times be the only available avenue for conceptualizing early interaction. In the following example, a young, depressed, and anxious woman entered treatment because she was contemplating becoming pregnant. She was certain that she wanted to have a child, but at the same time she feared she would be unsuccessful as a mother because her child would inevitably hate her or, at the very least, look down on her, and that any child born to her would inevitably be defective. The patient's depression and anxiety increased during the first several months of treatment as she reviewed a lifelong experience with a mother made dysfunctional through her addiction to sleeping pills and diet medications. The patient recalled always feeling angry and dismissive toward her mother, looking down on her, and being unable to turn to her for help of any kind. It was in the context of this deepening depression that the patient became pregnant. During her pregnancy, a new source of anger at her mother was elaborated: Her mother would most likely be as useless to her in the role of grandmother as she had been in her role as mother.

As Cramer (1992) suggests, the patient's negative experience of her therapist, the view of the therapist as similarly useless and ineffectual, worked against any hopes for the short-term intervention model that had initially been proposed by the patient. Instead, an old self with old other, patient–analyst relational configuration established itself in the treatment situation. That is, by virtue of being a woman, the analyst had become for the patient a strong retrieval cue of her mother, and a pattern similar to the pattern of relatedness in the maternal dyad was evoked in the analytic situation. The analyst understood that it was vitally important for the patient to remain in this old–old configuration, that she had no other experience to draw on in order to recategorize or experience the analyst differently, for example, as a maternal other who would be helpful, interested, concerned, and involved with her. The patient had no hope for the emergence of such a person in her life because such a person being connected to her was literally inconceivable for her. On her side, the analyst understood that in such a deep immersion within an old–old pattern, any intervention designed with the expectation of immediately initiating a different experience for the patient, successfully moving the patient into a new–new, or even an old–new, relational pattern was most likely futile, and, from the perspective developed here, not even desirable. We believe it is essential to allow the patient to remain sufficiently immersed in an old–old configuration, both because the patient cannot do otherwise and because the analyst requires the experience in the relationship if she is to come to know the patient's profound current needs and potent past traumas. In the case described here, over a period of 6 months in treatment, the analyst did indeed take on a new cast for this patient. The analyst's steadiness, reliability, attentiveness, indeed her very sobriety, appeared to have provided for this patient a new procedural experience in significant contrast to the traumatogenic, drug- and alcohol-induced procedural patterns long established with her mother, with this change in procedural experience predating in the patient declarative, insightful, self-reflective capacities. In this context, the patient's depression lifted slightly, and she gradually began to experience her analyst more positively, but remained deeply insecure about her own abilities. Hence an old–new relational configuration emerged, the analyst appearing as a novel, beneficial figure for the patient, but the patient continuing to suffer in old, familiar, painful ways.

The birth took place without incident, and 1 week later, much earlier than had been planned, the patient, feeling miserably depressed, was back with her analyst, spontaneously and without ceremony bringing her newborn daughter, Samantha, into the office with her. Thus began explicitly the mother–infant treatment situation that in actuality had been present from the beginning of the clinical work, but now the patient's trust in the analyst as one who could help in her mothering was made manifest. In this first postpartum session, the analyst responded with genuine delight at the unexpected arrival of the pair together, marveling at the baby's perfection and sharing in the pleasure of such an achievement. She commented upon Samantha's obvious calm and regulated demeanor, and noted as well how comfortable baby and mother seemed together. The patient responded with some surprise and even disbelief. She indicated that she feared something was wrong with her baby, and that something was wrong with the way she was with her baby, though she could identify nothing that could be seen to contribute to such fears. She was filled with questions about the meaning of her infant's responses to her, noting her discomfort that she could not possibly understand well enough her baby's communications. If Samantha cried, for example, while intuitively responding appropriately, she nevertheless perceived the cry as evidence of the baby's neither liking nor trusting her. If the baby slept, she anxiously wondered if this was because the baby was bored with her. She worried that the baby looked at others in preference to looking at her, based on the fact that the baby would turn away from her when someone else entered the room. She was certain that that turning away to look at others proved the baby would always like others better than the patient. All of these issues and many more were raised by the patient over the course of the next 6 months. A capacity to seek out the analyst as an informed, experienced woman, as a model for mothering, enhanced the evolving old–new pattern for this patient, based on her sense of feeling cared for and her observation that she could rely on her analyst's interest, competence, and positive regard. In turn, the analyst was able, in the context of the current ambience between them, to use her extensive knowledge of the patient's own past experiences to make crucial interpretive interventions that tied the mother–infant interactions to the mother's current and past relationship with her own mother.

In particular, the analyst connected her patient's fears about her baby not being able to like, appreciate, love, depend on, and trust her to the patient's sense of her mother's failures and her memories about how she had felt about her mother. A particular incident dating from first grade when her mother came to school for an open house, dressed sloppily, obviously stumbling and slurring her words, served as an emblematic symbol for such dysphoric feelings. Here the analyst helped the patient connect her sense of inadequacy and shame with her view of her mother when the patient was in first grade, and with the response she anticipated Samantha would have toward her. Thus, the analyst could interpret for the patient how she had experienced her baby as herself and herself as her mother.

Through this process, the patient was helped to move from a perception of Samantha as inevitably flawed by virtue of being her baby; to a perception of Samantha as perfect, but with Samantha experiencing her mother as defective; to, finally, a perception of her infant as lovable and loving, and herself as consummately worthy of her baby's love because of her competence and capacity to love her child and care for her needs. She was not yet at the point where she saw herself as lovable in her own right. For this reason, the treatment continued, with the mother–infant work being but a piece of a longer-term analysis.

We end this example with a consideration of the relational configuration apparent at this point in the treatment and the dimension of intimacy that was emergent. This was not yet a new–new relational configuration in its entirety, for although the patient was able to see herself as different in the context of her mothering, she was not yet able to see herself as worthy in all respects. Moreover, this patient was able to perceive her analyst as a self-transforming other and to perceive herself as a self-transforming other for her child. Interpersonal-sharing intimacy experiences were only beginning to emerge with her analyst and with her baby as well.

A mother–infant pair was referred when the baby was 8 months old by the baby's pediatrician for apparently intractable eating and sleeping disorders. The pediatrician had at first attempted to help the mother by instructing her in the Ferber (1985) technique in which the infant was allowed to cry for progressively longer periods of time until falling asleep. The mother's own method for encouraging sleep in her baby had been to offer the breast whenever the child cried, no matter how frequently the cries interrupted the parents' sleep, and then to allow the baby to sleep in the parents' bed, which did not help the sleeping and feeding disorders the mother was concerned about. Yet, although her own more permissive approach had not worked to regulate the baby's sleeping and feeding patterns, the mother found herself unable to comply with the pediatrician's advice and was feeling increasingly desperate. For this reason, she was referred to an analyst for help. The analyst asked the mother to bring her infant into the office with her, and in this first session the analyst was immediately impressed with the extraordinary frequency with which the baby, Lisa, demanded the breast and how automatically, and in fact apparently joyfully, the mother appeared to comply. Indeed, the mother spoke with pride about how attached Lisa was to her, and how well the breastfeeding had gone, but she noted as well that other infants in the play group she attended with Lisa seemed able to play for longer periods of time, actually allowing their mothers to engage in conversation with one another. She, in contrast, was required to be continuously engaged with taking care of Lisa.

Exploring the mother's history, it was easy to understand that the mother's pride was augmented by having her child so apparently securely attached, and herself so responsive to her child's needs. Her own mother had neglected her, leaving the patient in the care of numerous babysitters while the mother pursued her own career, putting her own needs ahead of those of her child. In contrast, and no doubt in response, the patient readily and happily sacrificed her own career in order to be always available to Lisa. The analyst, while fully appreciating the mother's capacities, was aware that this 8-month-old's requirements of her mother were more consistent with the requirements of a much younger infant. The analyst noted as well that any sign of frustration on Lisa's part was greeted with an offer of the breast, which the child readily accepted, so that the frequency of feeding was not only initiated by Lisa but initiated by her mother as well. In addition, from the beginning the analyst observed that the mother seemed not to understand Lisa's interest in exploratory play and the frustration that efforts on Lisa's part to achieve new developmental goals inevitably entailed. For example, when Lisa, crawling around the office in an initial exploratory move, was attracted by an object beyond her reach and reacted by crying and pointing, Lisa's mother neither facilitated Lisa's efforts to get to the object herself nor supplied an alternative attractive object. Instead, she picked Lisa up and brought her to her breast, saying, "Momma's here, my little girl. You need to suck." The analyst, remembering the mother's pride in her mothering capacities, and judging that this mother would interpret as criticism any direct observation from the analyst's perspective of what was happening, chose instead to distract both Lisa and her mother. She exclaimed, with authentic feeling, "Look how hard Lisa is trying and how curious she is! That's a sign of a secure and intelligent baby." At other times when Lisa reacted to being thwarted in her efforts, the analyst engaged Lisa in play, demonstrating that the baby's distress could be transformed into interest and pleasure in being led into a game with an other.

Through remarks and illustrations such as these, Lisa's mother began to distinguish the normal frustration and dysphoria involved in blocked exploration and play from signs of distress caused by hunger, signaling a need to be fed. This capacity to read more accurately the meanings of Lisa's discomfort, a capacity usually developed in the process of mothering, was interfered with in Lisa's mother by her fear of allowing Lisa to remain in a state of distress. She saw Lisa as herself, a child left all alone by her mother in overwhelming states of dysphoria, and focused on the attachment bond between herself and Lisa as the only means of allaying that fear. She saw sucking and feeding as the best means to secure the sense of connectedness, not being able to imagine a shared exploratory or play experience as being sufficiently salutary to address states of distress.

On her side, the analyst had some trepidation about not being more accurate in her descriptions to the patient of what she saw happening in the mother–infant dyad, and about not providing inter-pretation to the mother more directly. However, she determined upon reflection that she could accomplish her goal of helping the mother learn her child's needs through new, unreflected upon, experience rather than through hearing the analyst's observations and confronta-tions that might be interpreted as critical rather than helpful. Equally important, the analyst felt most intensely her own wishes to protect the mother, whom she saw as striving to do her best and as exhausting herself through her own efforts. She speculated that in approaching the mother in the way she devised, both Lisa's development and her mother's would be enhanced, and that both patients in her office would learn best in a positive ambience.

In fact, over the next 3 months of once-weekly treatment, the mother did learn to respond to her child's needs in a manner more accurately attuned to the particular requirements being expressed, and in the process was able to talk about some of her fears concerning leaving her child to cry alone at night, and her wish to help the child, by nursing her, avoid such fears as she herself had had when she was a child. The mother came to understand that she had not been in touch with her infant's proximal zone of development, but instead had kept the child linked to earlier modes of being comforted, soothed, and gratified. Through this process, the child's sleeping and eating patterns gradually became regulated and age appropriate, and her natural interest in exploration and play developed accordingly. For example, when Lisa awoke crying in the middle of the night, her mother could at times successfully soothe her back to sleep through rhythmic patting of her back and softly murmured expressions of love, avoiding the nursing ritual. The child not only developed a capacity to be regulated in this mutual-regulatory fashion, but learned as well to self regulate by ingesting greater amounts of food at each feeding, thereby lengthening the intervals between meals. Still later, Lisa, in the course of her normal development, began to acquire the capacity to soothe herself back to sleep upon awakening in the middle of the night, not requiring the active presence of the mother at all. Thus the child was helped to regain a normal developmental course. Daytime activities were also reflective of the mother's growing awareness of her child's varied needs. Heretofore whenever the child had cried for attention, the mother had responded by stopping all of her own activities in order to offer her breast. In treatment the mother acquired an ability to involve and interest her child in the activities of daily life to foster a mutuality of engagement that did not rest on feeding activities alone.

We understand this situation as one in which the mother was reliving with her child her own painful early experience, trying to undo her past through providing for her child what she had lacked. In the treatment situation, the analyst chose not to make this interpretation for several reasons. First, the mother's sense of herself as a competent maternal protective figure for her child was essential to both her own and her child's well-being. To question more openly the mother's interventions would have led the mother to feel shame, humiliation, and a sense of inadequacy, rather than her being able to experience the analyst and her comments as helpful.

Second, it seemed more advantageous to offer the kind of modeling that should have been available to the mother while she herself was growing up, available, that is, in the form of procedural memories from the past to draw on in the present for caregiving to her child. Thus, in the context of a new relationship with the analyst, strategies of caregiving were offered that represented alternative models to those in her own memory, allowing the mother to do more than repeat or reverse what she had experienced as a child. For the analyst to have chosen the alternative of interpreting the patient's behavior with her child might have risked ushering in an old–old relational configuration in which the patient would feel rejected and criticized, in effect deserted again by the person to whom she had turned for help, and the analyst would have been experienced as the rejecting, deserting mother of her past. As it was, a new–new relational configuration emerged, at the same time that insight into the meaning of her behavior with her child was garnered.

Part of what made the treatment so effective was the analyst's attitudes toward the mother, toward the dyad, and toward the process being initiated. The analyst had experienced a strong feeling of connection toward the mother, seeing her as willing and dedicated, admirable and competent to the extent that her experience would allow, and deserving of whatever aid the analyst could provide to her mothering process. The mother, on her part, had an immediate sense of trust and positive regard toward the analyst. This shared trust and regard created a strong bond between them, based on mutual respect and conviction about being responsive to the infant's needs, rather than abandoning the infant in her attempts at self-regulation, a strategy inherent in the Ferber (1985) method. The analyst also felt an immediate optimism about being effective with the mother–infant dyad, certain that she could help them move more effectively together on a developmental course. She saw herself as vitally connected to the mother, to the dyad, and to the process, an attitude that clearly facilitated implementation of mother–infant development.

Finally, a word about motivation. Here this mother had misperceived the meaning of her child's frustration in exploratory efforts, interpreting her child's needs whenever they were thwarted as requiring the type of attachment experience inherent in breastfeeding. This misperception involved two different aspects. First, the mother appeared to confuse frustration and distress in exploratory motivation with the motivation of hunger, and, second, the mother appeared unable to distinguish age-appropriate attachment experience in response to her infant's frustration and distress and was unable to provide a response that might have more effectively comforted her child without resulting in a concomitant sleep and feeding disregulation. Ideally the mother might have joined the child in play and facilitated the child's exploration of novel events and objects in the surround. In so doing, she might have expanded the range of exploratory opportunities she offered the child, moving into the arena of shared intimacy in playful activity. But even if she were correct in her assessment of her child as struggling with attachment longings, she might have offered something more age appropriate to fulfill these longings, such as soothing the child by holding the child on her lap. As it was, this mother had responded to only one motivational option, that of breastfeeding at any sign of distress, contributing thereby to the child's pattern of frequent nursing day and night. In consequence, feeding and sleep disregulations created a disruption in the family. These disregulations were addressed and resolved through a more attuned response to the child's needs.

This brings us back to our systems view in which motivation itself is a function of the experience with the caregiver in conjunction with the caregiving habits of the parental surround. Using this infant as an example, we can see physiological regulation, attachment, and exploration motives as all inextricably and intricately intertwined. If not for the interventions provided in the analytic work, one might predict a laying down of procedural patterns that might contribute to a later eating disorder in Lisa, or to disorders related to chronic separation anxiety.

At this point we will illustrate a parent–child developmental intervention within the context of an ongoing analysis. In this example, the mother began to find it progressively more difficult to be with her child as he became increasingly autonomous and out of her control. Patient and analyst had come to understand this experience in terms of the child's becoming for the patient an abusive and intrusive mother, modeled on the actual mother that the patient had experienced as a young child, a mother who in psychotic and alcoholic states would first escalate into frantic dancing, twirling, and singing and then, at times, erupt into enraged attacks on her child. On one occasion, the patient, who had been in analysis for about 6 months, brought her 14-month-old toddler, Josh, into the office with her because alternative care was not available. Josh began to explore the office, finding a doll house and a number of toys. As Josh became more and more stimulated in the context of this relatively novel scene, he became increasingly excited, pounding ever more vigorously with both hands on a leather hassock. His mother sat by, feeling in herself a mounting helplessness and fear of what she perceived as her child's frighteningly out-of-control behavior. In contrast, the analyst responded in a different way. He, with a broad smile of delight and acceptance, at first matched, with a patting motion and with a nodding of his head, the rhythm of Josh's excitement, and then automatically slowed the cadence of his patting and nodding to a more manageable pace, intoning at the same time in a soft and gentle manner, "O.K., O.K." The intervention, spontaneous as it was, served effectively to tone down the child's excitement, leaving him calmly continuing to play. But the more powerful effect was in the mother, who, observing this scene, understood for the first time on an affective level that her child was a little boy who could be helped to achieve a comfortable, pleasurable, and mutually regulated state, rather than being an unmanageable monster whose excitement and states of overstimulation foretold danger, all-too reminiscent of countless experiences with her mother. In this context, the analyst became a new maternal other for the patient, an other completely missing in the patient's past experience and an other who could be called on in the future to help regulate her own and her child's level of stimulation. A number of such instances followed of noninterpretive, unplanned, serendipitous interventions lived through in the analytic relationship, facilitated in their meliorative quality by the patient's positive relationship with her analyst. These interventions were not always experienced when the child was present, but were often based on interactions between patient and analyst alone.

In terms of relational configuration, the patient's experience of her analyst and herself transformed from an old–new to a new–new configuration as the patient began to experience herself, like the analyst, as more competent to regulate her anxiety and tension with her infant, with the effect of facilitating in the infant a new ability to regulate his levels of excitation. In terms of the dimension of intimacy, the analyst was experienced as a self-transforming other in this context, and, as in the previous example, the patient was helped to become a self-transforming other for her child.

The following example illustrates clinical work within the family–child surround, with a focus on how family stress affects the functioning of the child in the family, in this case a 2-year-old toddler, and then how that child's difficulties can be ameliorated through analytic intervention. Although in some cases it might be preferable to work with the child directly, this case exemplifies how intervention of any kind within the family can lead to meliorative changes, though the changes themselves are often unpredictable.

The parents brought their child, Mark, into treatment complaining that the child was easily distracted, irritable, and aggressive toward both parents, and had been identified by his toddler teacher as potentially hyperactive. The reasons for Mark's behavior seemed inexplicable to the parents, but they wondered whether genetic factors were at work because Mark's maternal uncle was manic–depressive. They were at a loss to see any other possible reasons for their child's symptoms. Because Mark was so young, and because neither mother nor father was identified as the specific therapeutic focus, the analyst decided to see the family together. At first nothing distinctive emerged. Mark was able to play in a concentrated fashion, remaining for the most part as a calm background to discussion between the parents and the analyst as Mark busied himself productively in the toy corner. However, one day in a session the parents found themselves in a bitter and explosive argument about money. What was remarkable about this event was that for the first time Mark exhibited in front of the analyst the behavior that the parents had initially complained of. He began to run aimlessly around the office, finally settling on the analyst's plant, which he had been told not to disturb. He tore off the leaves at random and with angry energy threw the dirt from the plant on the floor, an activity very like the things he had done at home and at school. The analyst himself had been surprised at the acrimony between the parents, as they had heretofore given the impression of relative harmony between them. He was surprised as well that their child's presence did not cause the parents to curtail their fighting in any way. Rather, they seemed at the moment oblivious to their toddler and to the effect they were apparently having on him.

The analyst, in pointing out, first, Mark's behavior and, second, what the parents had done that was perhaps related to that behavior, began a process of exploration, self- and mutual reflection, and an emergent self- and mutual regulation within the family system. What became clear was that when the parents fought, Mark responded with fragmentation, which was carried into the nursery school setting. The parents attempted to be more cognizant of the effects of their instability on Mark, trying to retain a calm in the surround, particularly on the mornings when Mark was taken to the toddler group. The effect of this work on Mark was dramatic. His behavior at home and at school improved immediately as the parents both stopped arguing in front of him and became generally more aware of the effects of their actions on him. It was fortunate that the marital relationship was solid and the parents' dedication to Mark was strong, so that they were able to address and resolve difficulties in the family system in just a few sessions. At this point, treatment continues only on an as-needed basis, and all talk of treatment for Mark in relation to incipient hyperactivity has long ago ceased. All in all, self-consolidation and consolidation of the attachment tie within the family has been strengthened.

We include this brief example to illustrate a few salient points. First, we want to note that with an infant or very young child, the developmental systems self psychology approach is particularly important because it opens up the possibility of entering into the family surround through any one or combination of its members. Second, when the child is very young, the problematic, procedurally mediated, emotional patterns may not be as fully entrenched and hence may be more available to change as new patterns are introduced, in this case the parents' learning to modulate and curb their arguments in order to avoid overstimulating their child. Here the analyst's role was to intervene early and, of course tactfully, to create a perturbation in an emerging family pattern of affect regulation in the realm of aggression. Intervention at this level facilitated a resumption of self-consolidation in Mark and consolidation of the attachment tie to his parents. It is important to note the connection between self-consolidation, secure attachment, and ability to regulate high levels of arousal, and that, in turn, self- and tie-to-other consolidation are compromised by an inability to regulate such affects. Third, we call attention to how hyperactivity is understood within our systems perspective. Although it is of course arguable that hyperactivity is best addressed as a dysfunction of the neurological organization of the child, from our vantage point hyperactivity may also be addressed from a systems approach in which multiple etiological factors are likely to play a role (Furman, 1996). In Mark's case, the hyperactivity could be conceptualized as his anxious response to family disruption, as identification with the aggressor, as reactive aggression to perceiving the parents' arguments as a threat to him, as self-regulatory efforts to cope with overstimulation, or as a simple affective resonance. Each of these conceptualizations could encompass as well some neurological predisposition, constitutional contribution, or set of temperamental factors.

Our point is that hyperactivity, like any other behavioral response, can be addressed effectively as a systems problem, whether that system is viewed on the level of the system self, system selfother, or system selfsurround. In terms of the latter, Furman has pointed out that the diagnosis and treatment of hyperactivity with Ritalin or a similar medication is 200 times more prevalent in the United States than in an area in Europe statistically comparable to the United States in terms of size and population. This finding represents a strong indication that diagnosis and treatment of hyperactivity are influenced by the environment, the system selfsurround.

PSYCHOANALYSIS OF THE PRESCHOOL- AND SCHOOL-AGE CHILD

Analytic work with the preschool- and school-age child may depend heavily on play to facilitate the child's expression of his or her inner world and to strengthen the relationship in the patient–analyst dyad. The symbolic aspect of play communicates where words alone are not sufficient, with the analyst either choosing to allow the play to continue unreflected on or choosing instead to interpret what possible meanings may be understood through the drama created between them.

Jordan, age 4, was brought into treatment because of his fears about sitting on the toilet, and because in nursery school it was noted that from being an outgoing, confident, and friendly child he had become rather suddenly excessively anxious, timid, and prone to daydreaming. Jordan had been upset for about 6 months following the loss of a 4-year-old friend of the family who had died suddenly of fulminating pneumonia. Because he had asked so many questions, he was told about the funeral and about how the child had been put into a hole in the ground. Having no clear concept of death, he had wondered how the little boy would eat, and whether he would be lonely and afraid of the dark. Despite the parents' explanations and attempts at reassurance, Jordan's anxiety continued. He seemed to formulate an unconscious belief that the toilet was like the grave, and that he could fall through the hole as his feces did and be flushed away to his death. He also worried that his penis and testicles might fall off when he sat on the toilet. He was aware of and could talk to his parents about the fear of losing his penis and testicles, but the idea about the toilet equaling the grave, the fear that his total body could be buried there, and the connection to his dead friend, was unavailable to him. Then after some months Jordan began to worry when his parents were absent that they would never return. At this point, because his anxieties had not diminished, he was brought into analysis.

When Jordan came to his first analytic hour, he had some difficulty leaving his mother. He had brought a toy bird with him. Once in the playroom, he spread bits of paper to create a trail that led back to the waiting room. Jordan explained that like the bird in "Hansel and Gretel," his toy bird could follow the crumbs and lead him back to his mother. In subsequent sessions, Jordan revealed his preoccupation with his dead friend. He pretended over and over to bury his analyst by covering him with paper and made believe he was feeding the analyst. He also made many drawings of a child in a grave, placing both food and drink there so that the child in the picture would not be hungry and thirsty. Finally, in yet another drawing, he pictured a grave with a ladder in it so that the person could climb out. The analyst talked with Jordan about the pictures, noting his worry about dead children, and complementing him on all the ways he had created to comfort the child and finally to rescue him. Thus the analyst chose not to confront Jordan with the finality of death, but rather went along with the child's age-appropriate self-protective strategies and attempts at mastery. Finally, the analyst made the connection for Jordan between his fear of the toilet and losing himself or parts of himself, and his fear of being buried without possibility of rescue, reassuring him that a lot of children have this worry, but that nothing like that could ever happen. It was shortly after this sequence of play and verbal intervention that Jordan was able once again to sit on the toilet without fear, not requiring, for the most part, an other to be close by while he defecated.

Although the death of the friend receded in his mind, separation fears remained prominent. For a time at the end of each week, Jordan would tie his analyst to his desk chair with Scotch tape, with the analyst explaining that Jordan wanted to make sure that his analyst would be there for him on Monday. Jordan responded indirectly by becoming even more enthusiastic about securing the analyst with additional quantities of Scotch tape. The play gradually diminished, only to recur when longer separations were imminent.

As fears of death and fears of separation subsided in Jordan's experience, a new theme became more prominent, concerning the wish to grow extremely tall and strong, like Superman, possessing large muscles, the ability to fly, and the ability to inspire awe in others. In an hour that most impressively demonstrated these newly emerging desires, Jordan used a puppet to eat the analyst's tie, explaining that this would make the puppet strong. Then, suddenly dropping the play with the puppet, Jordan himself began to play at eating the analyst's tie, teasingly but insistently. This allowed the analyst and Jordan to talk together about the tie's potent powers to make both the puppet, and Jordan, too, into men of importance, with, as Jordan said, "big muscles and everything." Play such as this seemed to herald Jordan's resumption of development, facilitated by his leaving behind the traumatic preoccupation that had interfered with it.

From our perspective, a new–new relational configuration had been established, with the analyst as a novel, powerful, understanding, and accepting other whose special abilities were there to be shared, with Jordan feeling newly able to grow and be strong, however impatiently and concretely (i.e., through eating the tie) he sought these changes. These views of the analyst were most likely like those he had begun to have earlier with his father, derailed by the trauma of the death of his friend, leaving Jordan with the feelings of unprotectedness and lack of safety with which he had begun the analysis. From our perspective, it was not useful to interpret, nor even to conceptualize, these now current, nonconflictual feelings with the analyst as a transference from the old, thwarted relationship with the father. Rather, in accordance with our framework, the capacities for positive relatedness had been integrated into Jordan's self, and were available for new expression at this time with the analyst as a novel other in his life. This is an instance of what we mean when we say that positive feelings stemming from good relationships in the past are not transference in our model but reflect a capacity integrated in the self to engage in similar good relationships in the present when they are available.

This same combination of play and verbal interactions can be seen in the case of Jenny, a 6-year-old girl who entered analysis because she had difficulty learning to read and because she was repeatedly caught stealing candy in school. Her young life had been characterized by intense jealousy and envy of her highly gifted, but deeply troubled brother, Jim, 2 years older than herself. Jim, from her vantage point, excelled in every way, including being loved far more than she was by her parents. In fact, the analyst's experience in her initial work with Jenny's parents seemed to make comprehensible Jenny's perspective. They were so involved with Jim that in the first several interviews with them, set up ostensibly to talk about Jenny's development, abilities, and

problems, Jenny's parents focused entirely on Jim's development, abilities, and problems, leaving Jenny out of their conversation in the same
way that Jenny felt they had left her out of family life.

Jenny entered into analysis with an immediate sense of envy that
her brother's analyst was far superior to her own. She complained to
her analyst that Dr. N. was much nicer, had more toys in his office,
and, in addition, would give Jim candy, just as the teachers gave him
candy for getting everything right in school. Jenny told her analyst
that she knew all of this was true because Jim told her so, including
how much better Dr. N. was than her doctor. Her analyst responded
that she knew Jim was always telling her things like that, telling her
that what he had was better than what she had, and that, in fact, he
was better than she was. Her analyst added that she knew also that
Jenny believed him when he told her that he was better and smarter
than she, that therefore Jenny felt there was no use in her trying to
compete with him. He was good in reading and she was not, so he was
given candy at school while she could only steal it. In fact, her analyst
told her, Jenny actually believed that girls were not supposed to do as
well as boys. Jenny looked surprised at all of this and responded by
saying that she had "something funny" to tell; her brother, who was
fat, slow, and lazy, could always beat her in a race even though she
knew that she could run much faster than he. When they raced, she
explained, Jim would hold his hand out to keep her from passing him,
and she had felt that were she to run around his arm and pass him up,
something bad would happen. Following this session, Jenny ran her
last race with Jim because she beat him and he refused ever to race
her again. This began Jenny's effort to do well in school. Only 2
months into treatment her teachers reported that they were pleased
with her progress, and Jenny said that reading aloud no longer made
her feel anxious. From this point forward, Jenny viewed her analyst as
a valuable person in her life. The analyst became a powerful protector,
in fact, a magical fairy godmother to Jenny's Cinderella, as the
following sequence illustrates.

The analyst became aware of Jenny's love for fairy tales around
the time when the child developed a virus. Jenny came into the office
lethargically, holding her collection of tales, saying she was too tired
to talk or play, and asked that her analyst read "Cinderella" to her. It
should be noted that the most satisfactory times Jenny had with her
mother were when they read stories together. Jenny listened to the
entire story without a word, and when the analyst finished, demanded
to hear it again. After that she would bring "Cinderella" with her from

time to time for the analyst to read whenever she felt herself slighted and misunderstood within her family. The story obviously reflected her sense of her situation at home. Jenny felt hopelessly criticized, unfavored, and unloved by her mother, demeaned and despised like a stepchild, whereas her brother, as she saw it, was catered to and adored despite the fact that he treated her and others so hatefully. She saw herself as aligned with her father, and as with the father in the tale, she saw him as too weak to protect her from the evil "stepmother" with whom she lived.

We want to make the point that there was no attempt to interpret either the meaning of the Cinderella story to Jenny, the use she made of it, or the view that Jenny had of the analyst as the fairy godmother who would magically make everything right. Instead, the idealization was allowed to continue, and the use of the story to configure the experience with her family went uninterrupted by interpretation. In our view interpretation is not always helpful in promoting the child's development, as will be discussed and illustrated further in our review of treatment with adolescents in the next chapter. We will just say here that at this point in the analysis an old–new constellation had already emerged in the analysis. The patient continued to feel at times sad and lonely in the old ways, but was already able to view the analyst in a new way, as helpful and protective, indeed, as possessing even magical qualities, which she felt were needed to alleviate her heretofore hopeless situation within a family that did not adequately perceive or meet her needs.

We include the case of Jenny also as a means of portraying and illustrating our developmental systems self psychology view of important phenomena that are subsumed under the umbrella of the Oedipus complex, focusing in our case example on castrated feelings in girls and castrating wishes toward boys, as will be illustrated below. But we want to note, first, our contention, contrary to that of many analysts, that the Oedipus complex is not a universal organizer of development, but rather is dependent for its emergence on experiences within the family constellation; and, second, that because one aspect of the complex is clearly demonstrated in a given patient, as we will illustrate in Jenny's case, all aspects of the complex need not also be present. Again, this is an individual matter based on lived experience. Referring back to Jordan and his playful eating of the analyst's tie, that engagement in play might easily be conceptualized as, in the main, a fellatio fantasy expressive of the oedipal child's wish to gain phallic power from the father in order to impregnate the mother by means of ingesting the father's penis and power. In contrast, the analyst in our example took the option not to interpret Jordan's wishes as expressed in play in this fashion, choosing rather to keep the interpretation more general in terms of the child's wish for grown-up masculine strength and status. This choice could be made because there was no evidence for the existence in this child of a fully developed oedipal constellation, and because the analyst did not assume automatically that the entire oedipal constellation must underlie any single aspect that is exhibited, nor that such aspects are always present in every child at this age and time in development. Again, the child and his or her experience in the family determine the nature of triadic relatedness and the relational patterns and symptoms that manifest clinically. The Oedipus complex is indeed a phenomenon that may be observed in treatment, and aspects of it may emerge in development, but, we would contend, it is by no means a *universal* organizer, in its full form, of every child's development. In our view, not all children unconsciously wish to have sexual intercourse with the parent of the opposite sex and experience murderous intent toward the parent of the same sex, nor do they fear that parent retaliating in kind both for their wishes and for their patricidal intent. And furthermore, the obligatory reverse of this complex—with sexual desires toward the parent of the same sex, and murderous feelings toward the parent of the opposite sex based on the child's innate bisexuality—also does not describe a universal organizer in child development.

To return to the case of Jenny, as already illustrated, her relationship with her brother was characterized by her feelings of anger, envy, and resentment, which feelings were reactive to his being physically and emotionally abusive to her in the context of a family in which his actions and attitudes went unchecked by the parents. She entered analysis in fear and awe of Jim, but once in treatment, became as bold and critical of him as he had always been of her, based on a sense of protection provided in the analytic relationship. That she saw herself as "castrated" at the beginning of the analysis—meaning that she lacked the penis her brother had, which symbolized not just for her but for the family as a whole his strength and superiority—was announced in the first picture she drew of herself with, as she said, "legs, so that she would not need crutches," her mother appearing in that same picture without legs at all. Jenny became preoccupied in her play with cutting out pictures of women from magazines and then cutting off their legs and mounting them on poster board. Also, she showed great concern about bodily injuries and scars.

One day Jenny brought a book into her session for her analyst to read, a child's version of *Moby Dick*. She said she did not know the story, but she had looked at the pictures, she knew the title, and she felt she had a pretty good idea of what it was about. The story was long and complicated, but she followed her analyst's reading with interest until quite suddenly she interrupted to ask if the analyst knew what a "dick" was, but then would say no more. Jenny and her analyst then talked about the peg leg of Captain Ahab and the peg arm of Captain Esmond, both injuries having been the result of actions of Moby Dick. Jenny then said that she felt the reason the story was called "Moby Dick" was because it was about a fish who did not really bite off people's dicks, but who did bite off things that looked like people's dicks, that is, their arms and legs.

In this context, in a later session Jenny brought in a poem she had written that had just won a prize in school. It began with the phrase, "A fish is a wish in the fierce dark sea." The analyst told her that the wonderful poem reminded her of the Moby Dick story they had read together. The analyst added that she knew she and Jenny had talked before about Jenny's terrible fear of something happening to her body and to the bodies of others, but the analyst wondered also if perhaps Jenny was afraid that she herself was like Moby Dick, that she had a fierce wish deeply buried inside of her that scared her, that she herself might want to scare and hurt others the way her brother had scared and hurt her. Jenny responded by announcing that what the analyst had said was ridiculous: "You have told me a lot of ridiculous things before, but this is the most ridiculous. Let's play." The analyst took from this strong, spontaneous response that no doubt she had said too much, more than Jenny was prepared to hear, and that the best thing she could do in this instance was to respond to Jenny's own assessment by agreeing to play instead of talk.

In retrospect, we would assert that it was an error to interrupt the play with unnecessary reflection, thereby disrupting an ongoing old–new relational experience with the protective fairy godmother analyst; the analyst with her disruptive, disturbing remark had become a frightening intrusive other, breaking the empathic, self-transforming intimate connection that had been so productively flourishing between them.

Jenny is a child who, in our view, clearly displayed symptoms ordinarily linked to the Oedipus complex, not because they were inevitable at this particular point in her development, but because the traumatic nature of her interactions in her family, wherein the boy was perceived to have power, took the form of penis envy, castration fear, and castration urges.

The following example concerns a family of refugees from Central America who had been referred to the treating analyst by the school for which the analyst consulted. The school had been concerned because the youngest child, Karen, age 7, had missed a great many schooldays, and even when present, she seemed unable to attend to the instruction offered. She would appear distracted, seemed afraid to go out to the playground at recess time, could not eat her lunch because she had stomach pains, and in general did not make contact with the other children or with her teacher.

The analyst, rather than seeing Karen alone, met with the entire family. The analyst began by asking about the home situation, and was certainly unprepared for the narrative that unfolded. The father began by describing the terror that existed for the family night and day in their current home environment. All windows facing the street had been boarded up by the father, and all family members slept on the floor in the back room of the house, by the father's report a set of tactics necessary to defend the family from dangers in the neighborhood, which included gang activity and drive-by shootings. In addition, the children were not allowed to play away from home after school, but instead had to come straight home in order to be safe and secure.

In describing this situation, the father broke into uncontrollable sobbing and began to shake. He talked about life at home in Central America, about friends and family who were incarcerated or killed in popular uprisings, and about his own sense of danger because of his politics. Leaving his country had become a necessity, he told the analyst tearfully, with the only means available being a dangerous and illicit passage first on land and then within a convoy of small boats. In attempting to talk about the circumstances of their voyage, the father suffered painful, frightening flashback experiences of the tragedy that occurred during their trip. The crew of his particular small boat held the family at gun point, took all of their belongings, raped some of the women, and beat up the men, but apparently left the children physically unharmed. The crew then deposited all of the passengers on a remote beach in Mexico.

The traumatic session just described, and the several sessions that followed, accomplished a great deal for the father, and for the family as a whole. The circumstances of his current living conditions could then be contextualized, revealing the extent to which life in the here and now was strongly influenced by the recent past, that his hypervigilance was registered as a necessity because events in Central America and on the voyage of escape had been an overwhelming trauma. The father was convinced that the trauma might be repeated at any time in their new dangerous environment, and that he had to prevent against all odds such a recurrence. Hence the boarded windows, the sleeping on the floor, the direct return from school, and the rules against playing away from home.

The analyst could now explain to the father that the shaking and crying he experienced represented flashback phenomena responsive to reliving the traumatic past in the present. Finally, the analyst could explore with the family as a whole what actions were required in their current circumstances for preservation of safety. All of this emerged in the family setting in which all family members were present. Specifically, the analyst could explore with the parents the actual character of the neighborhood, and how others living there managed. As it emerged, violence was more a rarity than a regular occurrence; children did walk to school and play at each others' houses after school, and families did not live behind barricades. The analyst of course was careful not to denigrate the experience of danger, nor to reassure the parents falsely against renewed danger, but rather attempted to assess with them the actual conditions in which they now lived.

Finally, in terms of the school's reason for referral, it became clear that Karen was afraid to go to school because, first of all, her family was afraid for her to leave the relative safety of the home for the dangers of the outside world, and, second, she herself was afraid to leave her family in the desperate circumstances that had been painted for her. The family's new awareness of the source of the fear allowed the past to remain past and the present to become present. The incipient school phobia in the child was immediately resolved, and the father's fears, although of course still present, were placed in context and became more manageable. The father was able to achieve a more consolidated self, less vulnerable to self-fragmenting flashbacks and more amenable to reflection. In turn, he was able to provide a more secure attachment for his daughter, who, in her turn, became less vulnerable to self-fragmentation and to self-shattering fears. Finally, the family as a whole became capable of a more realistic assessment of the current environment.

We are including this rather dramatic example of rapidly successful family treatment in order to illustrate once again several points. First, it serves as a stark illustration of the effects of life-threatening trauma on the individual; second, it reveals the degree to which the individual, in this case 7-year-old Karen, can at times only be understood in the context of the selfsurround; third, it shows the workings of the family as an interactive system, with each member affected by all others; and, fourth, it offers the developmental systems self psychology model as a vehicle for short-term treatment, short term because the analyst was immediately idealized as an effective authority who could bring into relief distinctions between past and present that had heretofore remained confused, and short term as well because the family itself was strong in its positive attachments to one another and existed within a state of goodwill and good feelings toward one another.

This next case illustrates long-term analysis with a 9-year-old boy referred for learning disabilities, and the difficulties that may ensue if both parents are not convinced that the treatment is essential to the child's well-being. It is commonplace in child treatment for one or both parents to begin to doubt its effectiveness, prematurely, from the analyst's perspective, when the treatment does not seem to them to be working, or, as in this case, when the treatment seems to create a new independence in the child, which is not always welcome to one or both parents. The analyst must take precautions to bring the parents along as the treatment progresses, a caution that cannot always be attended to effectively because of the particular dynamics in the family.

These latter circumstances were in evidence with the family of 9-year-old Timmy, who was referred for treatment by his educational therapist. She had originally evaluated Timmy to determine why he was unable to read or spell at levels appropriate either to his age or, as was shown by his performance on a standardized intelligence test. The educational therapist had been most impressed with Timmy's degree of anxiety as illustrated in the projective tests she administered. She wondered whether he might not be psychotic, or at the least what she had termed an incipient borderline personality with primitive defenses, based on Timmy's report that he at times heard voices in his head, and on her assessment of the stories he had constructed in a standardized projective test. It is important to note that Timmy's father was strongly opposed to Timmy's being in treatment and was suspicious of the treating analyst from the beginning, but because he was devoted to his son and sufficiently worried about him, he agreed to whatever help was deemed necessary by the educational therapist. The plan as it was initially construed was that Timmy be in analysis three times a week, leaving open the possibility of further educational therapy, and that any course of medication be held in abeyance until analysis alone was given a chance.

In the analyst's initial meeting with Timmy's parents, a few salient experiences in Timmy's life were revealed. First, the mother spoke of what she considered to be a key incident in Timmy's life occurring when he was 3. At a friend's birthday party, a clown appeared made up in a frightening disguise and suddenly, at one point in his performance, the clown made a very loud noise. Timmy screamed and cried inconsolably in abject terror, shook all over, and clung to his mother for several hours. After that experience he refused all parties, was horrified at Halloween, and found going away from home impossible. He therefore did not attend nursery school and was frightened through kindergarten, but by the time he reached first grade, he was able to be in school without obvious distress. Nevertheless, Timmy's mother continued to see him as fearful and easily put off by noise of any kind. A second incident remembered by his mother dated from when Timmy was 5, and he was strictly forbidden by his father in a firm tone from ever masturbating. Since that time, Timmy had been frightened of harm coming to his body, in particular to his genitals.

Timmy quickly developed a strong positive attachment to his female analyst, unlike the more ambivalent relationship established with his mother. This disparity in the boy's connection to his analyst as opposed to his mother was initially surprising to the analyst, but over the course of treatment she came to understand that the attachment to his mother, which had earlier in his life been more secure, had been influenced over time by what Timmy perceived to be his father's attitude, one of demeaning, patronizing superiority over his mother by virtue of her being a woman.

Not only was Timmy unable to keep from himself what he saw of his father's dismissive attitude toward his mother, but he also was subjected to his father's scorn whenever he dared to take her side, appeared to be too much like her, or, finally, appeared to be too close to her. In order to keep a tie to the father, he was forced to alter the tie to his mother. This attachment conflict was worsened because it was difficult for Timmy to maintain the view he sought to establish of his father as well as of his mother. He professed to see his father as ideal, without fault, and totally admirable, yet his father was loud, frightening, and shaming of any masculine weakness in his son, including Timmy's demonstrated need to be close to either parent. The attachment conflict experienced with his father was one in which the overt demand made of Timmy was for independence, but the covert demand was for total obeisance and submission to his father's need to be idealized by his son. These conflicts in attachment made it impossible for Timmy to consolidate a secure attachment bond with either parent, one attachment being incompatible with the other, and, in turn Timmy was unable to consolidate a solid sense of himself. This set of difficulties, appeared to lie behind the appearance of severe disturbance in the original diagnostic profile.

At first Timmy's use of his analyst was based exclusively on his explaining to her in depth who his father was, what his father felt, how his father functioned, and all of his father's thoughts. The effect of this experience for Timmy was to establish a connection to the analyst that permitted Timmy to feel secure at school and to be able to function and learn at an appropriate level for the first time. School difficulties ceased completely, as if by magic, and the need for educational therapy ceased as well. In fact, Timmy turned out to be a superior student, due in part, no doubt, to his cognitive abilities, but also to a new sense of safety and protectedness coming from the analyst.

For her part, the analyst was at first overwhelmed by this flood of information about the father, which allowed no interruption or commentary by her, but in time she came to understand that Timmy was showing her the hard, desperate work that went into sustaining a connection with and idealization of his father, risking no other commentary coming from the analyst that might not be in harmony with this ideal vision. After some time, the analyst noted to Timmy that she knew how much he admired his father, and how important his father was, not just in the world, at work, and with his admiring friends, but most centrally, how important his father was to Timmy. She added that she now knew so much about Timmy's father, because there was so much to know, but that there was no time for Timmy to say anything about himself, his feelings, his friends, or whatever else was important to him. At this point Timmy told his analyst about the voices in his head which told him how bad he was. Gradually a view of his father, and his father's loud, aggressive, angry, explosive voice, could be linked to the loud, aggressive, angry, explosive voice he heard in his head. He also began to talk about his mother, about how stupid and inadequate she was, and yet how he depended on her for love and care.

After some time, Timmy stopped talking about his father and his conflictual view of him so directly, and began to bring in comic books for the analyst and patient to read together. Timmy had a stack of favorite comics that depicted the lives of male superheroes, and each session he would require that his mother bring with him the entire collection, though Timmy and the analyst actually reviewed no more than a few pages of one of the books during any single session. The hours would go in a totally predictable manner: Timmy would begin by reading a few pages to the analyst drawn from a comic strip describing one or the other of his two comic heroes. One, Thor, was totally good, wise, ideal, fair, just, and incomparably strong; the other, the Hulk, was totally bad, stupid, mean, irascible, temperamental, demanding, and also strong, but not as strong as Thor. After an initial reading of one or two comic book pages, he would begin to compose, together with his analyst, his own comic strip in which the hero went from being totally good or bad to incorporating both good and bad elements. After months of this kind of activity, Timmy was able to take in the fact that the hero he created out of good and bad represented his father, who was, as he came to figure out, both good *and* bad.

At this point in treatment, Timmy for the first time began to confront his father, to differ with him, to demand to be recognized as himself, and to express openly and defiantly his regard and affection for his mother. Clearly the self-protective idealization of his father, so necessary for maintaining the tie to this brittle man, was receding as Timmy developed a stronger sense of himself and was more able to assert his right to be himself.

Unfortunately, his father, who had merely tolerated the treatment for 3 years because Timmy was doing better in ways that pleased the father and made him feel proud, that is, by excelling in school, decided unilaterally that it was time for treatment to stop. The analyst's relationship with the mother had always been quite good, and even had improved as time went on, but the father had only barely refrained from demeaning analysis and analyst, doing so for as long as he could and as long as it seemed to be to his son's advantage. With the new confrontation coming from his son, mild though it was in most respects, the father no longer felt the need to refrain from criticism. The analyst felt it was no longer possible for the analysis to continue without subjecting Timmy to the conflict of loyalties between maternal and paternal figures with which Timmy had first entered treatment. Indeed, there was already disruption in the family, with the father attempting to end the treatment by refusing to pay the analyst's charges, and the mother insisting that treatment go on and paying those charges herself. The analyst, weighing any potential gains that might ensue from further analytic work against the inevitable negative effects that would result were the analysis to continue against the father's will, concluded that Timmy required more than anything at this point a positive ambience at home. The analyst reasoned that even though some compliance and accommodation on Timmy's part would still be necessary, the stronger sense of self he had already attained, and his self-reflective capacity, would permit him to see clearly the reality at home and to know what he felt about it without fragmenting by once again splitting his understandings of his father, his mother, and himself into totally good and totally bad elements. These attainments, the analyst believed, were based on the secure attachment to her she hoped would sustain him even in her absence. Clearly the ending was less than ideal, with the attachment conflict with his parents more resolved but by no means laid to rest. The analyst was left with a frustrated sense of work interrupted, some doubts about her own effectiveness, and concern that she had erred in her judgment at the end.

Several years later the analyst received a letter from Timmy. Timmy wrote that he was doing well in school and had received early admission to a college of his choice. However, he chided the analyst for not having sufficiently protected him and their treatment. Because she had allowed him to confront his father as he had, the analysis had ended too soon. In the context of Timmy's criticism, the continued connection to the analyst, and the capacity to confront her, he revealed the consolidated self and consolidated attachment tie that showed development had proceeded satisfactorily. But Timmy's sense of loss of the analysis and the analyst, and loss of the security and safety it had promised, along with a loss in confidence in the analyst herself, were also revealed, adding to the analyst's concern that perhaps a different course of action would have been better, and that somehow she could have, should have, done more effective work with the father. In any case, follow-up, rare as it is, is always welcome, serving an invaluable purpose in improving our understanding of the process.

We conceptualize this patient as having had, at the beginning of treatment, a severely fragmented self resulting from an inability to consolidate either a solid sense of himself or a secure attachment tie to either parent. The initial idealization of the father was self-protective against recognition of the angry, fearful, irrational qualities he also saw in his father but could not allow himself to know. The

demeaning of his mother was similarly self-protective against a conviction that his father would not permit a more loving connection to
her. His fear of his loud and frightening father, represented in the
experience with the clown, was exacerbated by what he perceived to
be his father's threat to the integrity of his self, particularly his genitals.
His learning disability was secondary to his preoccupation with maintaining as best as possible the attachment ties to both parents.

At the beginning of treatment, an old–new configuration emerged
in which the analyst was viewed as a strong woman who actually had
the respect of both mother and father. In the safety of this situation,
Timmy was able to discover through his analyst's interpretive remarks
the nature and extent of his unconscious, self-protective idealization
strategy and the necessity for disavowing the more angry, threatening
father who lived as a disembodied voice within his head. In the
context of the new relation with the analyst and their mutual exploration of these matters, Timmy was able to consolidate a picture of his
father and himself as mixtures of good and bad, changing the split-off,
disavowed aspects of feelings toward his self and his father to a more
consolidated view in a new, intact, self-reflective self. A new–new
configuration became evident, reflective of Timmy's comfortable intimacy with the analyst and with himself. The evolution of this new
consolidated self enabled Timmy to endure the flawed separation from
his analyst, which surely carried with it elements of the original
trauma, that is, analyst as demeaned, inadequate mother. This capacity
in Timmy was supported by the fact that Timmy could in time write
his analyst of his disillusionment and disappointment with her, at the
same time that he reported himself as doing well. Thus, Timmy was
able to progress in his development despite the premature termination
and the vision of his analyst as flawed, and to do so without a repeated
vulnerability to fragmentation.

In the next chapter, we will continue our discussion of the clinical
situation across the lifespan, turning to adolescence.

CHAPTER EIGHT

The Clinical Situation across the Lifespan: Adolescence

A developmental systems self psychology, with the self defined as mindbrainbody, seems most appropriate in the treatment of adolescents, when the self is obviously influenced by many elements undergoing significant and rapid change. A nonlinear dynamic systems theory is required to grasp fully the multiplicity of factors involved. These factors include well-known and well-documented but nevertheless dramatic biological events such as hormonal, genital, and skeletal transformations; changes in cognitive capacities, metacognitive capacities, and capacities in symbolized and nonsymbolized memory systems; and an increase in the repertoire of self states specific to the adolescent period of life.

We would like to emphasize again, however, that all of these changes in the adolescent individual, as with the individual of any age, take place within the larger contexts of family and culture. Adolescence as a discrete period of development is actually an invention of Western culture, and continues to vary in terms of time of onset and offset from subculture to subculture within the Western world (Galatzer-Levy & Cohler, 1993).

As a part of this cultural view of adolescence, the salient role of the family in the development of the individual during this phase is traditionally perceived to be the facilitation of the adolescent's separation and individuation from the parental surround, a perspective in which separation and individuation are thus focal developmental concepts. In contrast with this view, we offer a developmental systems self psychology perspective that emphasizes a different role for the family, one in which security of attachment remains of central importance. From a nonlinear systems perspective, the connections among the elements of attachment, exploration, separation, and individuation are encompassed by the "secure base" concept of attachment theory, leading to the consolidated self and the consolidated self-with-other tie emphasized in our model. One crucial determinant of the patterns formed in the individual through the intertwining of these four elements is the nature of the environmental surround—whether responses to the individual are contingent or noncontingent, that is, whether the responses are based on the individual's needs and self states.

We can cite the infant research of Sander (1962) as an example of what is meant by contingent responsiveness related in particular to the achievement of individuation, which, like separation, attachment, and exploration, begins in early life. Sander contends that the infant becomes well regulated not as a result of an externally imposed schedule alone, but as a result of accurate responsiveness to the infant's internally based demands and signals. We use this model of the connection between the contingent response and the optimal attainment of the element of individuation as descriptive of the connection between such contingent responsiveness and the other elements, separation, attachment, and exploration. Moreover, the attainment of one element is intertwined with the others, so that greater individuation promotes a more effective capacity for separation, for exploration, and for healthy attachment, and all are encompassed by the concept of the secure base, as we indicated above.

As we understand and use these four elements, "separation" refers to the movement away from attachment figures; "individuation" refers to the sense of distinctiveness as an individual; "exploration" conveys a search for novelty and new experience and is positively related to safety and comfort in attachment; and "attachment" refers to the presence or absence of a secure base. Furthermore, this model and understanding of development applies across the life cycle, including our focus in this chapter, adolescence.

Particular issues in relation to separation, individuation, exploration, and attachment, potentially of importance at any stage of life, do take on foreground salience during the adolescent years. These include most prominently the new goals of heightened peer associations, finding pleasure and success in school and in the workplace, and creating a sexually evolved and evolving life of one's own, all arising within the context of an ongoing and safe connection to the family of origin.

We contend, moreover, that where such an ongoing and safe connection is not available, the adolescent years may become riddled by conflict, the disturbed adolescent suffering from insecure attachment. The professional literature on this topic is somewhat inconsistent. The older psychoanalytic literature had stressed the norm of difficulty, turmoil, and states of rebellion in adolescence. This view was challenged first by Offer's research (1969), and more recently by Galatzer-Levy and Cohler (1993), who all postulate that adolescence as a stage of life is often traversed without undue upset. Most recently, Hamburg (1997) presented a perspective that confronts such sanguine expectations for the adolescent period. Hamburg pointed out that adolescent children from ages 10 to 15 are faced with inordinate external pressures, for example, to use drugs and weapons and to engage in premature, unprotected sexual behavior. He contends that some are unable to resolve conflict without violence, and that many are depressed, with about one-third having considered at one time or another the possibility of suicide. Hamburg concludes, "By age 17, about one-quarter of all adolescents have engaged in behaviors that are harmful to themselves and others, such as getting pregnant, using drugs, taking part in antisocial activity, and failing in school. Altogether, nearly half of American adolescents are at high or moderate risk of seriously damaging their life choices" (p. 7).

How do we reconcile these different conceptualizations of adolescence as a phase that may be lived through easily versus adolescence as a phase most often fraught with great difficulty? From our perspective, the way adolescence is negotiated by the individual is highly correlated with the maintenance of a secure attachment to the family and the evolution of a concomitant hope for the future, wherein success and happiness are seen as likely attainments. Therefore, we see this responsibility for healthy outcome as belonging to the family as a whole: to help the adolescent find new ways to relate within the family unit that enhance his or her secure attachment and at the same time enhance phase-appropriate separation, individuation, and exploration experiences. For example, Fonagy, Steele, Steele, Moran, and Higgitt (1991) contend that the parents' continued appropriate responsiveness to the developing individual's attachment needs is significantly connected to the individual's attainment of the capacity for self-reflective awareness, permitting an awareness of the subjectivity of the other as well as one's own. This is particularly relevant for consideration here, as the capacity for self-reflection is heightened in adolescence through the development of cognition into formal operations (Piaget & Inhelder, 1969).* Other attachment theorists (e.g., Stern, 1995; Main & Goldwyn, 1985; Bruner, 1990) connect parental responsiveness leading to a secure base with the elaboration of the capacity for self-narrative formation, a capacity that also facilitates an understanding of the other's narratives. Both of these abilities are elaborated during adolescence. These combined achievements heighten the focus within the securely attached family on the achievement of interpersonal-sharing intimacy between the adolescent and other family members. The adolescent attains an enhanced capacity to appreciate others, as well as himself or herself, as persons in their own right.

One aspect of this evolution in relating effectively and maturely within the family is the expanded role of mentorship assumed by the parents (Bloch, 1995). Mentorship is built on the earlier roles parents assume in coaching the team, bringing the child to the adult workplace, helping with homework and other school projects, and, even earlier, making and implementing play dates and constructing Halloween costumes. Ideally, mentorship goes on into the offspring's own middle age, when parenting is expanded to grandparenting (Cath, 1985). The role of others in the family as mentors for the adolescent individual does not end, then, but remains that of providing both encouragement and support. Just as what Piaget (1962, cited in Uzgiris, 1973) refers to as "deferred imitation," the earliest ability of the toddler to imitate in their absence actions performed by others, heralds the independent capacity to do and be, always and inevitably embedded in the lived relationship with others, so in adolescence, role identification and role reversal occur with the same effort toward competence and mastery. The child who was coached by others comes to be, as an adolescent, a coach for others.

---

*Although we refer to Piaget and Inhelder (1969), for a more complete contemporary discussion of cognitive development, see Galatzer-Levy and Cohler (1993). Cognition is not treated formally as a separate capacity because, from a systems understanding, such cognitive capacities are complexly intertwined with constitutional and experiential factors, and not separable from affect and self state. However, there is at a macrolevel a broad progression from nonsymbolic to symbolic to progressively more abstract thought and self-narrative formation. Traditionally, the mature phase of cognitive development is formal operations, when the individual's ability to imagine a future, to reverse operations mentally, and to think abstractly is in full sway. As we have already shown, such capacities are inseparable from attachment, self integration, self-consolidation, and in general, the capacity to manage one's transference, that is, the freedom from suffusion of the present by the past.

Just as these interpersonal-sharing capacities for intimacy evolve in the adolescent as a member of his or her family, individuation also evolves with an expansion beyond family life, toward the development of peer-group relationships and toward a continuing maturation of private aspects of the self. An inner fantasy world comes to provide functional capacities and resources for the individual. Both of these developments—expansion of intimate relationships and maturation of the capacity for privacy—represent continuations of, rather than distinctions from, what went before and both are achieved on the basis of a secure attachment.

The movement beyond the family is widely recognized in Western culture and widely written about in the psychoanalytic literature. We will focus our brief discussion on the sexual aspect of that movement because biological changes during adolescence bring sexuality to the foreground as a central, strong motivational force essentially for the first time in the child's life. We contend that when sexuality is a strong motivational force earlier in life, it is correlated with neglect or more active abuse suffered by the child in the environment. Although some children may appear to desire sexual contact and to seek it out, these efforts are best understood as wishes for sensual experiences with a loved other. In a less healthy family setting, such approaches may be more openly sexual, and may represent either sexualized attachment or an enactment of abuse, turning passive into active. Moreover, when a child of any age, including but not limited to the adolescent, approaches a parent with affectionate physicality, that parent's most appropriate response is to understand and accept the ascendant sensuality or affectionate need in the child, at the same time that the primary role as attachment figure for the child is kept central. In this experience, the child will be protected from crippling conflict, but the child's ongoing capacity for sensual sexual expression with an appropriate other outside the intimate family circle is preeminently preserved. We are in agreement with Mark Erikson (1993) who makes the general observation, based on studies of the Kibbutz organization in Israel and the Simpua marriage in Asia, that secure attachment is an important protective factor against child's sexual abuse from any quarter.

We see it as helpful to recognize that although wishes for sensuality, including genital sensuality, are often openly expressed by the infant, toddler, and even the young school-age child, such expressions are not likely to be, as Kohut (1977, 1984) had postulated, breakdown products of a fragmenting self, but are manifestations of a healthily consolidated self. We are in agreement, as we indicated in the last chapter, with Kohut's (1984) larger point that pathological oedipal conflict is not inevitable; its pathological expression can be considerably mitigated or avoided altogether in a family in which the child's attachment needs are kept as a primary focus and are met with contingent responsiveness. The 4-year-old girl who dresses, however seductively, in Mother's clothing does not really wish to be treated by Father as if she were his sexual partner and, in any case, is not best served by being admired as such. Her role as cherished little girl should be preserved. The school-age girl who wishes to dress, not in Mother's clothes, but like Mother, again is not well served when she is treated as the sexual person she is striving so hard to emulate. And in adolescence, the now-pubescent girl who hugs her father in her wish to be close does not wish to be responded to by him actively and overtly as seductively attractive. The father and mother function in all periods of childhood as secure bases from which the child and growing adolescent can explore in safety and security, free to turn outward and to turn inward. All of this is of utmost importance in adolescence where sexuality and sensuality are in the foreground of subjective self-experience as well as in the foreground of other, non-experiential, nonsubjective aspects of the self, such as changes in growth hormone levels and testosterone and estrogen levels. These latter, nonexperiential, nonsubjective changes influence in slow and subtle ways sexual maturation, adding weight to the more subjectively (and intersubjectively, interpersonally, and objectively) perceived transformations in the adolescent. It is imperative that the youngster be understood and helped to find appropriate expression for attendant compelling sexual needs and wishes.

This brings us to the topic of individuation and private aspects of the self in adolescence, also in its ascendance during this time when sexuality is so prominent. Privacy does not begin in adolescence; much fantasy play in the school-age child can be private and is increasingly so as the growing individual becomes less and less reliant on external props for fantasy elaboration. There is an increasing capacity in the child and the young adolescent to be able to fantasize by manipulating ideas and symbols internally without concrete representation. As sexual changes enter into the child's self system, sexual stimulation, masturbation or its equivalent, and accompanying fantasy emerge as new phenomena to be dealt with. Friedman (1988) hypothesizes, based on considerable research on male development, that a specific sexual fantasy formation arises spontaneously in the adolescent boy during masturbation, reflecting, tagging, and signaling the sexual orientation that has emerged, influencing his future course as either heterosexual male, homosexual male, or bisexual male, a finding that conforms to our own clinical experience. To our knowledge, similar research has not yet been done in the female population, but our clinical work, limited as it is, does not suggest that such an eruption of spontaneous and specific fantasy tagging sexual orientation in adolescence does occur in females, although we speculate that homosexual masturbatory fantasies may indicate some potential for lesbian or bisexual interest. In any case, with both male and female patients, the sexual fantasy arising at that age period is of great significance as a new element in the self system. With girls and boys, sexual fantasies can serve and express attachment needs and mastery of heightened desire, but what is most often present and prominent is the use of sexual fantasy to serve requirements for normal growth and development and for adapting to, or mastering conflict evoked by, the new awareness of mature genital sexuality.

This self-reflective awareness of the self as a sexual being is conducive to the attainment of privacy. From early on, the child embedded in a family that respects cultural and developmental norms of privacy increasingly wants to maintain privacy within that family and in the peer group in regard to sexual matters, beginning with the wish to keep private bodily functions, including the wish to cover up sexual parts in front of others. Where parents' attitudes about privacy do not respond to the expressed needs and wishes of their children in this regard, the child may feel either invaded or intruded upon, may become exhibitionistic in the extreme, or may respond by feeling something is wrong with him or her for wishing to maintain a personal life, as if keeping something hidden reveals something aberrant about the self.

The growing capacity to maintain a private world in which ideas are manipulated in thought alone stands in contrast to the younger child's need to play out ideas through action, toys, or tangible, symbol-laden props. In the fantasy life of the adolescent, such props may or may not continue to play a significant role, but in general, there is an increasing capacity in the adolescent for formal operations and abstract thought, permitting more of one's fantasy life and thought to be kept private, so that more choice is available to share or not share one's personal world. More particularly, the evolution of formal operations contributes to the adolescent's ability to conceptualize something that has never happened, creates a new potential for imagining both the future and abstractions that can never exist in the real world. We contend that this new ability for formal operational thought, together with the earlier and ongoing capacity for self-narrative formation, permits the adolescent who is securely attached to imagine a new, different, expanded personal world, to imagine that things can be different and better for himself or herself and can be rendered as such by him or her. We connect to secure attachment this capacity for imagining a better future for the self, just as Fonagy, Steele, Moran, and Higgitt (1991) connected the capacity for telling a coherent autobiographical narrative. Moreover, we believe that this ability for self-reflective metacognition, which emerges so strongly in normal adolescence, is of great importance clinically.

TWO ADOLESCENT CASE EXAMPLES

This leads us to two adolescent case examples, both of whom were referred for treatment by psychiatrists who were impressed that their symptoms met the diagnostic criteria for overanxious disorder of childhood according to the fourth edition of the *Diagnostic and Statistical Manual of Mental Disorders* (DSM-IV, 300.02; American Psychiatric Association, 1994). Although a consideration of DSM-IV criteria is not ordinarily paramount in psychoanalytic thought, we have chosen to discuss the issue here for two reasons. First, we are often required to think in these terms in order to interact with colleagues around issues of diagnosis, medication, and insurance coverage, as these issues may well be relevant in a psychoanalytic treatment. It may provide as well a means to communicate with other mental health professions about our patients and the best use of additional forms of intervention, such as medication, hospitalization, and behavioral and cognitive treatment modalities. Second, and perhaps more important from a developmental systems self psychology perspective, psychiatric and psychoanalytic concepts are often integratable and in fact may prove to be mutually enriching. Such diagnostic criteria can be useful and important to an understanding of a patient on a nomothetic, nondynamic level of observation, which stands in contrast to the more idiographic, dynamic level of observation pertinent to the psychoanalytic perspective. The two levels taken together in a systems view, which highlights the linearity of DSM-IV features, integrated with the nonlinearity of psychoanalytic understanding, may offer a fuller perspective on the patient.

Charlie

The first case we will present involves a boy just entering puberty, and the second a boy in midadolescence. We will attempt to demonstrate in these case illustrations many of the points we have just made regarding adolescence, particularly the analytic relationship and the analytic interventions that are important in this period of developmental progression.

Charlie, a charming, socially engaging boy of 11, who was just on the cusp of puberty, was referred for analytic treatment by the priest who served as principal of the parochial school he attended. The referral was based on his teachers' and parents' concerns regarding his preoccupation with explosives and explosions. They had all noted, also with some anxiety, Charlie's uneasiness regarding the bodily changes that were just beginning to emerge into his conscious awareness, this uneasiness being picked up in classroom conversation by his teachers. His parents in particular worried that if their son were so preoccupied now with explosives, what might he grow up to be? They pictured an emergent Unabomber or, even more likely, an IRA terrorist and were looking for some kind of reassurance, either direct or indirect, that their child would grow up to be normal. Unfortunately, this expectation was not met either from the school or from the two previous consultations, one with a conscientious psychopharmacologist who recommended medication for the child's anxiety disorder and the other with a dedicated child analyst who, apparently taking the symptom as literally as the parents and school had done, perceived it as an expression of uncontained, unfettered, murderous hostility and recommended urgently that the child get intensive psychoanalytic treatment.

The parents, even more confused and troubled, then took the boy to another psychoanalyst whose assessment differed considerably. After only one session, based on his experience of Charlie's self state, this analyst had the distinct impression of a child playing with the *metaphor* of explosiveness, rather than one who was preoccupied with its concrete actuality. He based this assessment, rapid as it was, on several factors. First was his clinical feel that he was in the company of a robust, vital, and optimistic young person, bursting with an energy only moderately impeded by his anxiety, which was indeed substantial. He did not see the degree of anger and hostility postulated by the first analyst, and could only imagine that it was inferred by that analyst predicated on the symptom itself. Second, based on his inquiry,

Charlie was able to tell him that the explosive fantasy was kept to his imagination and play with toy bombs purchased at the toy store. He was not, as other young, apparently more troubled and alienated adolescent patients the analyst had worked with previously, seriously experimenting with chemicals intended for actual vandalism. Third, Charlie seemed securely attached to his parents, as well as to his teachers and peers. He expressed friendly feelings toward others and was not preoccupied with hostile, destructive fantasies directed at specific persons.

We would like at this point to digress a moment to address questions we anticipate concerning what might be seen as the obvious oedipal nature of Charlie's preoccupation with explosions. Our approach, as indicated before, incorporates an alertness to any oedipal presentations appearing either directly or in a disguised manner. However, we do not assume *a priori* the existence of active pathological oedipal concerns in an 11-year-old just because he has reached the point of adolescence. Nor do we assume that explosion is inevitably a metaphor for sexual or aggressive drive derivatives. Finally, we do not assume that if one sees the patient more often, four or five times a week, then the "true" oedipal nature of the pathology will emerge. It might emerge, but not inevitably.

To return to the clinical situation, the analyst's attitude toward Charlie, based on his perception of the basically healthy, though overly anxious, restless, and keyed-up, self state manifested by him, was a reassurance to the parents, who themselves were then able to understand that the explosion preoccupation symbolized the rapid development of his self, his mindbrainbody in transition. However, treatment seemed indicated for Charlie, despite the fact that his self state was largely a response to age-expectable bodily changes. The degree of his anxious, restless, and keyed-up state, together with his vulnerability to irritable moods in relation to his mother and father, indicated that his development, in danger of being compromised, would be facilitated by analysis. Indeed, the constellation of symptoms he manifested did appear to meet diagnostic criteria for DSM-IV overanxious disorder of childhood just as the referring psychiatrist had indicated. The analyst believed that medication should not be the first resort because of the developmental attainments already manifest in Charlie, and the solid relationship he appeared to have with his family. Therefore, the analyst opted to begin with therapy alone, hoping that the relationship with him would act to calm and contain both Charlie and his parents. We will describe something of the treatment in order to illustrate both the developmental progression of this patient into full adolescence and the therapeutic interventions that seemed called for as the treatment progressed.

To begin with, Charlie was seen only once a week, so as not to strengthen the link, in the parents' mind, between frequency of treatment and severity of illness. These parents had been traumatized by the suggestion of analysis four times per week and by the previous analyst's ominous tone, so the current analyst did not feel it would be helpful to Charlie to enhance the parents' susceptibility to viewing him as pathologically compromised. Moreover, the analyst's own feeling was that too great a frequency would interfere with and disrupt Charlie's relatively healthy connectedness to his peers and afterschool activities. Although two or three times a week would have been the analyst's initial suggestion, on balance it seemed wiser to begin with less and to increase only if necessary and then only judiciously. Also, he wanted to reserve the right to see the parents as required. Although seeing parents may be disruptive to a patient of this age, this concern must be taken in context, and here, the parents were eager for and clearly needed the help afforded by regular contact. Charlie did not express the need for greater privacy from his parents, though the analyst did sense that this was coming soon. The whole dynamic system needs to be taken into consideration in introducing a powerful new element, such as analytic treatment, for one of its members.

Overall, the experience with Charlie over the first several months of treatment did confirm the analyst's sense that Charlie was enacting and attempting to master his age-appropriate apprehensions about his changing body in the context of a family that was not fully in touch with the meaning and significance to him of these self-state changes. His parents had misread, influenced by the strong suggestion of the first psychoanalyst, Charlie's preoccupations as indicative solely of anger and destructiveness, rather than comprehending and appreciating his use of dramatic play and sports in ways that were adaptive, socially acceptable, and socially acclaimed. His parents' own anxiety about Charlie's development and their failure to recognize Charlie's new self state as an expression of his concern about biological change contributed to their responding in a less than contingent way to Charlie's signals.

In these early months, the analyst also came to understand that although Charlie had always much admired his father's strength and position in the world, more recently he had become disillusioned with him, which undermined his ability to accept his father's reassurance at the very time when he so deeply needed this heretofore soothing and self-regulating tie. His mother retained her steady presence with him, but could not fully compensate for the disillusionment with his father. All in all, Charlie was suffering from a subtle but nevertheless effective diminishment of the positive regard he was able to feel coming from both parents, and they in turn felt less secure in their ability to be of use to him. The analyst came to understand this in various ways, principally through Charlie's ability to talk directly about his concerns in this regard.

In one session, for example, Charlie entered the office limping from the effects of a sprained ankle. He anxiously related that he felt his father had minimized the injury, encouraging him to just walk on it and it would be all right. He added, somewhat cynically, that his father saw himself as "the doctor" in the house. The ankle was painful and appeared swollen. The analyst acknowledged the swelling, saying that he could understand Charlie's worry about it despite his father's reassurances. But he also noted to Charlie that his father had had much experience with such injuries. Thus the analyst acknowledged consciously though indirectly that each had a valid perspective, opting to help Charlie perceive his father's benign, although somewhat misattuned, attempt to be supportive rather than to resonate and empathize solely with Charlie's concern. The analyst had been aware of his own self state wherein the opportunity to examine his patient's ankle activated a longing to practice physical medicine once again, along with his sense that the injury perhaps might have benefited from more treatment than Charlie's father had indicated. But because there was enough question in his own mind, and he wished not to undermine Charlie's father's stature, he chose the route of helping to repair the bond between patient and father, while at the same time affirming Charlie's distress.

This example is included because it contains subtle but important considerations. On the one hand, there was the emergent idealization of the analyst, and on the other, the threat to Charlie's connection to his father based on disillusionment with him. Had the analyst assessed the connection between Charlie and his father as irremediable, he might have chosen to address only Charlie's perspective, interpreting his disappointment and sense of hopelessness about relying on his father. As it was, the analyst felt Charlie's attachment to his father was enhanced by the direction the analyst chose to take. The treatment process, including interaction with the parents, provided opportunity to help both father and son understand one another's perspectives, so that interpersonal-sharing intimacy could be enhanced, that is, the capacity of each to see the other and value the other as an individual in his own right. Both individuation and attachment were thus addressed in an intersubjective process.

At this point we will return to our earlier discussion of the role of interpretation in clinical work, now as it pertains in work with the adolescent patient, distinguishing it from other interventions. In adolescence the growing individual becomes increasingly capable of self-reflection, at the same time that the requirement for play and external props to facilitate thought and expression is diminishing. Interpretation can play an important role in accelerating this developmental course. We define interpretation rather broadly as the *verbal* or other *semiotically encoded* assistance offered by the analyst with a view toward enhancement of the patient's self-reflective capacity. This broadly defined view of interpretation will be illustrated in the following discussion of the clinical work with Charlie.

Charlie had consumed the first several months of his treatment talking about all the ways in which one might blow up buildings, especially buildings that housed authorities, like the White House, the IRS, the Church, and his Catholic school. The fourth of July could be, he speculated, a big holiday for him, as he considered how to get around regulations that prohibited the purchase of fireworks. Charlie concluded that if only he were older and able to drive, he could get to remote places where such purchases were possible. He told the analyst that he loved the movies, and he apparently ranked them according to the degree and quality of explosions they portrayed. He was skillful in demonstrating through bodily expression how, in slow motion, an explosion took place on the screen, acting out with sensual intensity both the explosion itself and the people who were affected by it, either by being damaged in the explosion or by being successful in their escape. Alongside of this preoccupation was his dramatic demonstration of advanced abilities in volleyball, having progressed in that sport to club level. Serving, punching, leaping, both in natural speed and slow motion, Charlie acted out a volleyball scene, just as he had acted out the explosives scene.

The analyst did not choose to interpret, except in the most vague terms, either Charlie's physical activity or his conflicts about growing up. That is, the analyst did not ask him to reflect upon what might lie behind his pronouncements or his activity or what their meaning to him might be, in order to build his *self-reflective* capacities. The analyst's activities *were* designed, however, to promote Charlie's *self-*

awareness within a positive, accepting, self-regulating ambience. The analyst's reasoning in this regard was complex. First, the analyst viewed Charlie's activity and ongoing commentary not as primarily self-protective, not as designed to hide or contain more crucial meanings, but as self-expression that still required props, toys, and activity for its achievement. In other words, the analyst perceived his patient as telling about himself in all the ways available to him, expressing whatever his subjective concerns were in the moment in a manner that also revealed his attempts at mastery. Second, the analyst reasoned that interpretation of this material, attempting to create in Charlie more self-reflective awareness, would run the risk of embarrassing him by making him feel transparent to the analyst, and thus would most likely have interrupted the ongoing experience of talking with a feeling of safety and in a mode of comfortable intimacy and sharing. These are aspects of analysis that we view as essential, and at times as more salient to the analytic process and to the development of the individual than the process and effects of interpretation itself. The value of revealing to Charlie the analyst's speculations about possible defended-against unconscious content and conflict formation was dubious in contrast to the value of establishing a secure attachment that would enhance self-awareness, but which would leave the more direct, verbally encoded enhancement of self-reflection for another time. In our view, the establishment of such a secure attachment base promotes a more *spontaneous* self-reflective capacity, a readiness to become aware of and to share with the analyst heretofore less consciously available conflict and content. Third, the analyst knew from Charlie's mother, because he had broached these topics with her, that Charlie was at times aware of his fears of bodily change, not being able to "bulk up," and of sexual excitement, and also of the shame and humiliation attendant on not being prepared as a sexual adult to deal with girls. The analyst opted to respect Charlie's choice of whom to be intimate with, and in what manner that intimacy was to be made manifest. By following Charlie's lead, the analyst was offering Charlie a relationship in which he felt neither transparent nor alone, but where he could decide for himself how much of himself to share. Fourth, we believe that interpretation of any speculated, defended-against contents would have disrupted Charlie's attempts to self-regulate in an ongoing fashion his burgeoning sense of physical power and sexuality, and his attempts to sustain the analyst as an idealized other. The patient's need seemed to be more in the nature of engaging the analyst in his preoccupations, enjoying the analyst's admiration of his prowess, and being soothed by the reassurance attendant on having an ally who respected and admired him and who proffered an ongoing positive regard. Interpretation, in our view, is but one element in a successful analysis. In the case that follows, we will demonstrate a situation in which interpretation is more salient to the ongoing work.

Roger

Roger, age 14, had been referred for treatment by the secondary school he attended because his grades had plummeted and he seemed restless and distracted in class. He was referred first to a psychopharmacologist because the school suspected attention-deficit/hyperactivity disorder and then, following that physician's diagnosis of overanxious disorder of childhood, and his recommendation for medication, the parents opted to seek a second opinion from an analyst. As with Charlie, a diagnosis was made, a recommendation for medication was given, and a second opinion was sought. The treatment was begun with Roger without the use of drugs as Roger himself and his parents as well did not wish medication to be used.

Roger agreed to see the second analyst, and on his first visits mainly expressed his profound disillusionment with his parents, which had begun much earlier in his life but which had come to a peak because the arguments that had pervaded family life were now culminating in a possible decision to divorce. Although Roger had always been anxious, with chronic sleep disturbance and some school phobia in elementary school, he had done well in his studies, but now he found himself unable to concentrate. When he tried to work he would feel upset and restless, unable to focus his thoughts, and would turn to television and to his CD collection in order to bring himself some calm and self-containment. His presentation also focused on themes of hopelessness tinged with cynicism about the adult world, and a certainty that his own life as an adult would be no different than either his parents' life, which seemed to him soaked in misery, or his own state at present. Moreover, he told the analyst, no one cared about anyone but himself, so that although he had accepted the school's referral, he did not imagine that it was an expression of concern or caring. Rather, he saw it as an effort to make the school run smoothly and to keep their profits up. Roger was undecided as to whether he would leave home and the incessant arguing in his family and go to live with an aunt in another city. He had actually written to this aunt and she had agreed to have him if he chose to follow through. The analyst's response on these early visits was to listen to her patient, and to acknowledge the core of truth in his presentation, especially as it applied to his own life at present with parents who were indeed unavailable to him because of their marital problems. She then proposed that perhaps by talking more about it together, they could come to understand why he, unlike her, felt life could never be any different. Although Roger remained dubious, after several sessions with her he agreed to meet twice a week.

In the analyst's assessment, Roger was a lonely adolescent whose defensive use of cynicism both expressed his core of hopelessness that life could ever get better and protected him from being disappointed and disillusioned again. Although he seemed depressed, the analyst was more impressed by his anxiety, which kept him restless and distracted. Earlier he had been fearful of leaving home for school and the current wish to move away from home to live with his aunt was seen by the analyst as similarly defensive against fear of being left once again by his unavailable parents. The aunt herself had not been important in his life, but at least she had done nothing to hurt him, and she was willing to take him in.

A significant intervention well into the treatment process was that of pointing out to Roger the analyst's sense that his wish to leave home was primarily a protection against awareness of his longing to be close to and protected by his parents. This interpretation was followed by conveying to Roger the analyst's sense that Roger felt it was his parents who wished to have him leave home, and that Roger had protected himself further by preempting them and adopting the desire as his own. This did not preclude, the analyst told him, the fact that indeed he might be happier in another family, but that for right now it appeared that his wish to leave home had also to do with the fear of being rejected once again. Roger was able to recognize the validity of these interpretations, directed as they were toward increasing his self-reflection in the moment as well as to promoting increased self-reflective capacities. Equally important was the information conveyed to the analyst by Roger's response: He did seem to her to be at a point in his development where interpretation could be valuable to ongoing therapeutic process.

As work continued, and Roger developed a more secure attachment to his analyst based on his comfort within the relationship, he became able to express the feeling that perhaps the analyst could not be trusted any more than his parents or the people at school could. In the sessions Roger would at first feel understood as he described a circumstance in his life, or would experience a sense of being cared for when the analyst responded to his hunger by offering him food or when she laughed at his jokes with genuine appreciation. There would be in those moments some apparent relief of anxiety in him, but this was followed by a fear that this sense of safety could not last, and he would once again retreat to cynicism. He finally told the analyst that he feared she only expressed empathy for profit; in other words, he was afraid that she was no more concerned with him, and cared no more for him, than the school when they originally referred him. How could he know, he asked, whether the analyst was an adult he could really trust or one who only pretended to be trustworthy? She addressed this important question by telling him that he could only know by assessing her responses to him as either authentic or not. Roger was able to remind himself that his analyst did actually seem to like him, and to care about and remember what he had said. He noted also that she was willing to see him at odd hours, hours that he perceived to be outside of her ordinary schedule. But in the context of this mutual reflection on their relationship, Roger noted that however trustworthy the analyst might be, she was not really helpful to him, because nothing was getting any better in his family. He finally challenged her with the assertion that of course she would agree with him while only he was present with her, but that it would be different were his parents there too. This line of argument led the analyst to wonder with Roger whether he felt it might be helpful to include his parents in a session. Prior to this time, Roger had steadfastly refused to have his parents come in, despite their willingness to do so, but now, it seemed, he had garnered enough trust in his analyst that he was willing to take the risk, a trust in her disguised by the sarcastic assertion that she would certainly not have the courage of her convictions, even assuming they were honest convictions.

The analyst recognized that in one sense, Roger was correct, though she felt that he assumed incorrect motives on her part. She did worry about being confrontative with his parents, that they would remove him from her care if they felt that she was disruptive to family unity. However, because Roger had shown some improvement in school and in other areas of his life, and also because she had talked to his parents on the phone about Roger, and had felt their real concern for him as well as appreciation for his improvement, on balance she did not worry too much about seeing them in a session with Roger.

The family and analyst did all meet together, and the analyst opened the session by expressing her concern about two areas in their family life. First she worried that there was so much fighting between the parents without apparent regard for Roger's obvious anxiety, despite the fact that his symptoms were often exacerbated by such family arguments. Although they were somewhat aware of the connection between the arguments and Roger's distress, apparently the parents' own difficulties precluded their ability to curb their acrimony in front of him. As a second concern expressed in the family meeting, the analyst described her sense that Roger feared the parents actually wanted him to leave home, and that Roger defended himself against that perception by insisting it was his own desire. The analyst added that this insight helped her and Roger to understand Roger's anxiety about being deserted, which contributed to his inability to sleep and to concentrate. The parents were able to listen and to hear, so that from this point on, they became more aware of their effect on Roger, but just as importantly, Roger was able to see the analyst as more concerned with him, and less concerned with a selfishly motivated need for profit. A secure attachment to the analyst was facilitated.

These changes in Roger, and concomitant changes in the relationship with the analyst, allowed the pair to focus on Roger's sense of hopelessness, his sense that things could never get better for him. He began to move from self-awareness to an increased capacity for self-reflection, and with this capacity came an ability to imagine himself in the future, and to imagine the possibility of a future for himself that would be better than the present. Along with this emergent attainment of hope and optimism came a new interest in peers, school activities, and dating.

At this point we will address the theoretical and clinical issues that guide our thinking about Roger and the course of his treatment. First, in contrast to the work with Charlie, Roger was at a point in his development on entering treatment where the interaction with his analyst was basically conducted as a verbal exchange. Roger could use words and did not require the use of toys, play, or props to express himself. Second, we would characterize Roger's attachment to his parents as ambivalent, and it was this ambivalent attachment that had presented as anxiety and as the various self-protective strategies adopted to cope with that anxiety. As we conceptualize it, Roger had as a small child suffered from school phobia (included in DSM-IV Category 309.21, separation anxiety disorder), and then as an adolescent, he presented with a more generalized anxiety disorder (DSM-IV Category 300.02, including overanxious disorder of childhood).

In the context of the analytic situation, what emerged in the interaction with his analyst was a Category C ambivalent attachment. From our developmental systems self psychology perspective, we conceptualize that Roger's insecure attachment to his parents interfered with his self-awareness as well as with the more advanced development of his self-reflective capacities and ability to utilize formal operations to the point where he could envision himself in the future. The achievement of a secure attachment relationship with his analyst facilitated not only the above capacities, but also the capacity to self-regulate and thereby modulate his own anxious self states. Through the analyst's interactions with Roger's parents, which were aimed at ameliorating disconnections within the family, the parents were helped to respond to Roger's needs more contingently, an experience that over time permitted the establishment of a secure attachment bond to both parents as well.

Other aspects of adolescent attainment also developed in Roger during the course of analysis in the context of his secure relatedness with his analyst. Roger, who had been socially isolated during his latency and early teen years, began, as we have stated, to expand his connections to his peers. In this context, Roger also revealed an interest in girls for the first time and could talk about his fears in this regard. While he freely discussed his hesitation to ask girls out, based on a concern that he would be rejected, and openly displayed a need for reassurance and affirmation, Roger at the same time expressed his familiar anxiety that all the talk would do no good, and that he would never achieve a life in which he loved and was loved by an other. At this point in the analysis, then, Roger was facing with his analyst old fears now interpreted and understood, in the context of newly acquired abilities to hope for a different and better experience for himself. In such a context, affirmation and reassurance coming from the analyst were vitally important. These affirmations and reassurances, the heightened self-reflection stemming from accurately timed and empathically resonant interpretations, and, finally, the experience of meeting with his parents and his analyst in a session that clearly addressed his needs, together constituted for Roger the positive new experience that he required to further his development.

We will address briefly at this point the trajectory of developmental progression as it is reflected in these two adolescent patients. Roger entered into analysis with only ambivalent attachment patterns available to him. Thus, he could and did reach out with anticipation of positive response at times, but there was also always available a pattern

suggesting the inevitability of disappointment in any attached relationship. Hence, when he evoked a perception of his analyst as
empathic only for profit, that the analyst demonstrated no more real
concern for him than either the school officials or his parents, the
other side of the ambivalent attachment was in the foreground, and
an old self with old other, patient–analyst relational configuration was
emergent in the dyad. Roger saw himself and his analyst at that
moment in the same hopeless, neglected, lonely, traumatized way that
he had experienced himself in relationship to significant traumatogenic others in the past and in the present, from time to time. Put
simply, the analyst was assimilated into the old, familiar pattern—self
in interaction with traumatogenic other—possibly the only pattern as
yet available to Roger or, alternatively, the only pattern he could safely
allow at the moment.

In time, with the analyst continuing to listen, to understand and
respond contingently, and to sympathize, the patient, although still
caught in old ways, incapable of feeling differently about himself and
without hope for his future, began nevertheless to experience the
analyst as a person different from the neglectful, unavailable others in
his past. This was especially marked when the analyst met with his
family, showing consistency in her attitudes and her faith in him.
Thus, with Roger, there was an extended period in the treatment
during which he viewed his analyst as wanting to help him and capable
of understanding him, able to put Roger's situation into words that
conveyed that wish to help and that understanding. However, Roger
remained without hope that he could ever be happy or could ever
achieve a new and better life for himself where he would be loved and
respected as himself by others, until, beginning with the family
meeting, he was able to experience in his analyst more than the good
intentions, which after all he had already experienced, however
inconsistently, with his parents. So, while Roger continued to assimi-
late his current self on the model of the past in terms of how it was
to be in interaction with an other to whom he looked for care, he
could finally see that the analyst was a distinctive, unique other in
that particular relational configuration, and he developed a beginning
appreciation for and accommodation to a positive new other in his
life. Finally, at present, a beginning sense of himself as a new and
different person is also emerging, the effect of a new secure attachment
to his analyst. Also, as a consequence, he is more able to hope and
plan for the future, and to take chances in interpersonal relationships
that go beyond his analyst.

In terms of the dimension of intimacy that described their relationship, Roger alternated between experiencing his analyst as a self-transforming other, especially as the analyst was required to respond over a long period of time contingently to Roger's needs (e.g., in terms of being flexible about hours, making food available, and exploring his unique interests and activities) and, less impressively, as an interpersonal-sharing other, particularly in the context of supplying desired information about her life, including her thoughts, interests, and desires, whenever Roger himself solicited such understanding.

Turning to the other example, Charlie represented an instance in which, from our perspective, a patient did not enter treatment with old self with old other transference proclivities. In contrast to the assessment of the first analyst Charlie had seen, the analyst in our case example did not perceive the boy as suffering from dysphoric and explosive aggression based on early experiences with destructive aggression predominating in relationship to his parents. Instead, Charlie's preoccupation with explosions was viewed primarily as an age-appropriate, self-expansive, self-regulating phenomenon used by Charlie unconsciously to contend with rapid and destabilizing adolescent physical and emotional change. His normal response was heightened by his parents' anxiety regarding Charlie's physical and mental changes so consistent with his newly emergent adolescent self. They were unable to contain and regulate either their own or his worry in this regard, and their own exaggerated concern was greatly exacerbated by the first analyst's alarm and view of Charlie as pathological.

Understanding and communicating to Charlie from the perspective of his preoccupations being relatively healthy, age-appropriate responses to adolescent change right from the beginning of the analytic work allowed a new self with new other configuration to emerge early in the analytic relationship. As we have indicated throughout this book, it is not necessary for an analysis to begin with an old–old relationship experience. Moreover, we believe that this example illustrates the multipotentiality of relational configurations that a given analysis might assume. In this instance, because the treating analyst saw Charlie as being on a course of normal development but being made anxious by the dire expectations of his parents and by the dire predictions of the first evaluating analyst, the treating analyst was able to respond to Charlie in a way that reduced the anxiety, ushering in a new–new relational configuration, which has maintained itself throughout the course of the analysis to date. The case clearly illustrates the significant role of the analyst as a codeterminer of the course of analysis, and in particular, as a codeterminer of the sequences in the trajectory of developmental progression. Finally, it shows the importance of match between patient and analyst contributing significantly to outcome. We contend, although without any evidence for it, that this boy did better with this analyst then he might have done with the analyst who had originally evaluated him. This contention is based on our conviction that positive new experience leads to the best developmental result.

CHAPTER NINE

The Clinical Situation across the Lifespan: Adulthood

In this final chapter, we will discuss two patients, each of whom presented for analysis with a diagnosis of DSM-IV major depression. For the reasons we cited in the previous chapter, we incorporate this psychiatric terminology in our consideration of these depressed women. We are often required to think in these terms in order to interact with colleagues around issues of diagnosis, medication, and insurance coverage, as these issues may well be relevant in a psychoanalytic treatment. From a nonlinear dynamic systems perspective, psychiatric and psychoanalytic concepts can be integrated and may prove to be mutually enriching.

There are nine symptoms recognized as diagnostic for this category of illness in DSM-IV, five or more of which must be present in the patient for the diagnosis to be made, with either depressed mood or loss of interest or pleasure in life always required as a part of the symptom repertoire. The symptoms include depressed mood most days, and most of the day; markedly diminished interest or pleasure in all activity; significant weight loss or weight gain; insomnia or hypersomnia; psychomotor agitation or retardation; fatigue or loss of energy; feelings of worthlessness or excessive guilt; diminished ability to think or concentrate; and recurrent thoughts of death, suicidal ideation, or suicidal attempt.

TWO ADULT CASE EXAMPLES

The two patients we will describe below each met these criteria for major depression, and although each had been diagnosed as needing medication, both, for different reasons, were medication resistant. They were therefore treated psychoanalytically, without antidepressants, using our model. From this point of view, the context and process of observation, which, of necessity, is highly interactive and vitally intersubjective and interpersonal, becomes of greatest importance. Although the two patients were understood to present as diagnostically similar to one another, with similar symptomatology, once engaged within the context of an analytic relationship the perspective changed, and the elaborated picture that emerged demonstrated substantial differences between them. We hope to make the point that although these two patients, whom we will call Emily and Theresa, presented with the same diagnosis, their illnesses emerging in the clinical situation were actually quite different from one another, with their differences introducing etiological distinctions of importance. In turn, treatment interventions emerged that were unique to each particular patient. This is a perspective in which the diagnosis, the understanding of etiology, and the treatment itself are all conceptualized as components of a nonlinear dynamic systems process leading in a rather unpredictable fashion to an always individualistic outcome.

Emily

Emily, the first patient, introduced herself by describing herself as feeling utterly without interest in going on living. Were it not for her daughter, she said, she would undoubtedly have taken her own life long ago; only her sense of responsibility for her child kept her tied to life. Were she to kill herself, she reasoned, she would be risking inflicting on her child the same unbearable sense of emptiness and abandonment that she herself had felt for as long as she could remember. Emily also complained of intolerable sleepiness, compulsive overeating without appetite, lack of energy, and feelings of intense loneliness. The second of three children, Emily described her parents as singularly without personality or affect. She had few discrete memories of either of them stemming from her childhood, and when she thought of them at the time what came to her mind was absence, void, a profound distance from life, in fact, deadness. They lived in another city, rarely visited, and seldom established phone contact, but any communication with them at all created in Emily feelings of being alone in a vacuum. She described how her father, on his infrequent visits to her home, would on arrival walk into her house, kiss her and her daughter perfunctorily in greeting, and immediately turn to television, retreating from any conversation, even though he had not seen her or his granddaughter for many months. Her mother would sit quietly in the background, content to wait for someone to amuse her. When Emily was still a child, her parents would travel every summer back to their home town, and to their parents, leaving her alone with her brother who was 3 years older. The two children would have to fend for themselves for weeks at a time, depending on family friends and neighbors for whatever comfort they could not find within themselves. The brother, Sam, was of great importance to Emily. As she described the situation, he was the only one in her life who had ever made her feel safe. He would be the one to talk to her, to defend her against others, and to teach her what he knew of life. Without any insight into the meaning of the term, Emily would call him "Brommy," an obvious contraction of brother and mommy and an unconscious allusion to his double meaning in her life. The sense of safety gained in relation to him was devastatingly altered when she was 13 and Sam contracted osteomyelitis secondary to an ill-treated broken elbow, resulting, after a 2-year period, in his arm being amputated. Also when she was 13, her younger sibling was born. As a consequence of these developments, Emily's teenage years with her family were experienced as even more vacant and ungratifying than her earlier childhood had been, but it was during this time that she began to excel in academics and to be recognized in the world outside her family as highly gifted.

During college Emily met her husband-to-be. Like her, he was an outstanding achiever and like her brother, he made her feel safe and protected. They became lovers and best friends, and enjoyed many activities and experiences together, but nevertheless, Emily remained relatively low-key. They went on to marry right out of college and entered into a highly successful artistic enterprise together, and their marriage appeared to work extremely well until their baby was born. Becoming a mother required for Emily an intense focus on her daughter. She was conscious of her own efforts to be present with the child, to be the mother she herself had never had, a mother deeply responsive to and highly involved with her child. The effort demanded was considerable, absorbing all of her energy, inasmuch as she had no model to draw on for optimal parenting. She would be aware of herself trying to be herself with her child, standing back from the immediate experience to criticize her own efforts, despite the fact that, from all outward indications, her mothering was certainly more than adequate. What stood out for her was that her husband was unable to facilitate this process. He could neither admire her efforts nor supplement them.

Rather, he complained bitterly of her unavailability to him and mourned the loss of their close friendship and erotic love, which seemed to have been foreclosed by the presence of a child in their lives. By the time Emily entered analysis, she and her husband were already close to separating.

Emily had been referred for treatment by the competent psychopharmacologist she had consulted several years before regarding her depression. She presented to him her history of lifelong dysphoria, describing parents and siblings who were also depressed. Her two siblings take the same antidepressant, Zoloft, and experienced considerable relief from that medication. Understandably, Emily's psychopharmacologist began by prescribing Zoloft for her, only to be followed by numerous other psychopharmacological products, alone and in combination, all of which failed for one reason or another. None made her feel better, and most made her feel considerably worse due to their side effects. It was with some impatience, obviously feeling at the end of his psychopharmacological rope, that the psychiatrist described this patient as one of a group who seem somehow "unwilling" to allow medication to work, an attitude that he may have unconsciously and nondeliberately conveyed to her. Later, he reassured both patient and analyst that there were always new medications to try, and indeed, try them she did once in psychoanalysis, but with the same effects. Every failure made her feel worse about herself: as she experienced it, she could not even do medication right.

Emily entered analysis with little hope; in fact, she described herself as *without* any hope, fearful that, as with the medication, having no hope meant getting no help. Although this attitude has changed very little in her several years of analysis, she has continued to come to her appointments consistently and on time, and when business takes her out of town, she seeks to set up phone sessions. A sample vignette taken from her second year of analysis provides a sense of what it is like for the analyst to be with Emily.

In this particular session, after an initial greeting, Emily came in, sank into her chair, averted her head, and remained silent for some time. This was a most familiar experience, and the analyst had learned to sit quietly with her for as long as it took. Emily had helped the analyst to understand that this sequence was the most effective way to aid her in starting to feel a semblance of connection to the analyst, and then to herself, within the mutual silence. Emily's capacity to feel the analyst's presence and to anticipate her analyst's response without great aversion was a new attainment in relationship to an other, an outgrowth of the analytic work signifying a nascent attachment and an emergent trust and comfort in the analyst's presence. The analyst saw the relationship as beginning to fill in, though just barely, the sense of emptiness that had plagued the patient for so long a time. He speculated that this patient's relationship with both parents was that of distance, absence, and neglect, rather than of harshness and criticism directed against Emily. He speculated further, and interpreted to his patient, that Emily learned as a small child to explain to herself her parents' lack of interest in her in terms of Emily's own sense of badness, that Emily probably came to believe that she was worthless and unlovable or else there would be no way for her to understand her parents' neither attending to her nor loving her. She had therefore come to expect with profound conviction that no one would ever have any interest in her, or even want to hear her talk, an unconscious organizing pattern that explained why it had taken so much time for Emily to believe that the analyst really did want to hear what she had to say, which in fact was so.

In this new context of a beginning attachment, Emily was able to speak less hesitantly, less haltingly, and with less shame, and in this particular session she could finally begin to talk without prompting. She told her analyst that she was very sleepy and was having a hard time, harder than usual, staying awake, and that this had been true that day even when trying to do her work. What analyst and patient had discovered thus far in treatment was that ordinarily working provided the only time when Emily felt alive and involved, not self-consciously self-critical and self-demeaning, not withdrawn from contact with whatever she was doing and whomever she was with. Ordinarily she could work extremely well and was noted for her ability to concentrate on and complete a creative task with inordinate speed, but that day, she told her analyst, she was unable to connect at all with the task at hand. The analyst noted to himself that her speech was slowed, even more than usual, reminding him of the psychomotor retardation with which she had presented originally. He noted also that she seemed bored with what she was saying, which he perceived as another way in which she had returned to earlier modes of being with him, born of a certainty that he would be bored with her. As the analyst watched and waited for Emily's next words, she began to rub her cheeks and temples in a harsh and tortuous way, kneading her forehead with troubled hands, which he again recognized from the past and had come to understand as a self-regulatory effort on her part designed to attain some sense of aliveness. Then, slowly, she began to speak.

She told the analyst about two experiences from the day before that served to convince her, yet again, that no one wanted to respond to her needs, even when meeting her needs would benefit *them*, even though she was willing to pay, and pay well, for their services. One experience concerned her attempt to hire a house painter, and the other concerned her search for a particular piece of Early American furniture. In both instances, the individuals concerned failed to show interest in providing the service Emily desired. The analyst responded by acknowledging the possibility that both the house painter and the antique furniture dealer were uninterested in working with her, but he noted also that she frequently experienced herself as unable to get what she wanted from others. Even when she wanted something from him, he reminded her, she still felt convinced that she would not be able to convey her desires in a way that would engage his interest or make him feel like responding to her. The analyst told her that it made him think of past instances in the analysis when she would convey to him a certainty that he would not change an appointment time for her when she needed it, or call her when she was away from the city, though these fears were not expressed in words. At those times, the analyst told her, he would recognize a particular tone in her voice that expressed to him her doubt and hesitation, and he would observe a physical movement away from him that could have been read as a wish to disengage rather than to engage. He quickly assured her that he, of course, understood that it was her feeling that she did not *deserve* his responsiveness that created the particular constellation of behavior, but, he added, it made him wonder now whether others who did not know her nor understand her so well would be misled, would misread her move to disengage as disinterest, and her appearance of hesitancy as withdrawal. The analyst asked her, could both of these men, the antique furniture dealer and the house painter, have similarly misread her intentions? Emily hesitated, and the analyst noted a slight edge of discomfort, leading him to respond spontaneously with a story of his own. He told her that there was a time early in his career when he had been mysteriously unable to cash valid checks in the supermarket, whereas his wife would have no difficulty in the same situation with the same check. The analyst then told her that they had discovered together that there was something about his manner, something completely out of his awareness, that would telegraph to the store manager a sense of lack of entitlement. The story reached his patient, they both laughed, and she visibly relaxed, her heavy mood apparently alleviated for that moment.

It is easy enough to understand in retrospect the analyst's spontaneous self-revelation as an effort to reduce the nascent, emergent
shame Emily had demonstrated at being faced with an unwitting,
nonconscious communication of her private feelings. He had already
learned with this patient that addressing her shame directly would
destroy her very tenuous, always threatened connection to him, so he
had spontaneously chosen a different path. His story permitted her to
reconnect to him without feeling shame, reassured that the analyst
was neither blaming her nor viewing her as inadequate. Instead they
could enjoy the shared humanity of this remembered experience from
his own life, at the same time that the experience might aid Emily to
reclaim and integrate something of the unconscious, nonconscious,
nonverbal aspect of herself.

We believe that an important component of this nonverbal aspect
of the self is procedural memory, memory that is laid down nonsym-
bolically, encoded in cognitive, affective, or physical patterning, im-
plicit rather than explicit, and without language mediation. We
postulate that patient and analyst were co-constructing together new
procedural pathways, as well as symbolically mediated understandings
that could protect Emily from the familiar trough of shame and blame,
moving her into a development-promoting positive new experience of
self-esteem-enhancing connectedness and pleasurable interpersonal-
sharing intimacy with an other.

We hope we have made clear in this rather pedestrian, undramatic
example some important points regarding this particular patient. First,
Emily, however biologically compromised she might be, suffered from
an empty depression associated with actual lived experiences of emotional deprivation and neglect. Second, the treatment to this point
had provided positive new experiences, which were both procedurally
and declaratively encoded, that is, encoded in action patterns without
concomitant symbolic representation, and encoded in a semiotic,
symbolic fashion. These experiences included, first, opportunities for
optimal self-regulation arising in the context of an intimate attachment with a self-transforming other; second, occasions for an intimate
attachment with an interpersonal-sharing other, in this example particularly as regulating shame and feelings of aloneness; third, possibilities for the development of self-awareness and of self- and mutual-
reflective capacities; and fourth, opportunities to co-construct a verbal
self-narrative that helped to explain herself to herself, and that
contributed to self-consolidation and consolidation of the tie to the
other.

Theresa

Theresa originally came for brief psychotherapy to help with problems she was experiencing in raising her infant son, who at the time was 3 months of age. The difficulties she described in this postpartum setting included self-doubts about her competence as a parent, and strong feelings of guilt concerning her maternal function-ing, which extended to anxiety about doing her child harm through her inability to be a constant and calm mother. She expressed as well suicidal ideation and suffered from disregulated eating and sleeping, accompanied by insomnia, weight loss, psychomotor agitation, trouble in concentrating, and feelings of deep hopelessness. Thus, according to DSM-IV, on first appearance this patient more than met the criteria for major depression.

Theresa's husband was a high-energy, high-powered business ex-ecutive, and expected from his wife the same kind of competence and efficiency that he always demanded of himself. His business took him away from home a great deal, leaving Theresa to care for her child alone, and he felt quite impatient with his wife's obvious distress over being left with responsibility for their son.

If there had been any question about the gravity of Theresa's depression, it was removed when 1 month into treatment she made a serious suicide attempt, which, fortunately, could be handled promptly in an emergency room setting. The analyst, of course, despite her patient's strong unwillingness, considered antidepressant medication right from the start, and her suicide attempt only heightened the analyst's sense that medication was indeed essential. She insisted that Theresa see a psychopharmacologist, which she did. Theresa experi-enced any medication that was tried as extremely unsettling, and she refused to maintain the prescribed regime. Exploring the problem with Theresa led to a puzzling response on her part: She explained that any medication felt to her like an intrusion into the functioning of her body, a frightening takeover by something foreign and outside of herself. Nothing further could be discerned at that time, and the analyst felt she could do no more than to respect her patient's decision. The alternative course agreed upon was to intensify treatment to five times per week, which the analyst hoped would contain her distress, and in any case would provide the optimal conditions in which to explore the puzzling picture.

A few months into the analysis, as Theresa was getting up to leave the office, she felt suddenly faint and dizzy, leading to an exploration for the first time in some detail of her eating habits. Theresa, while slender, did not appear anorectic. The analyst knew that her depression had resulted in some weight loss, but until this time she was unaware of Theresa's efforts to regulate her intake of food, efforts at physiological regulation that resulted in significant periods during which she would avoid eating anything. At that moment in treatment, however, Theresa was able to tell the analyst that the dizziness was a direct result of a current period of subjecting herself to semistarvation. This unpredicted development in the analysis created considerable anxiety in the analyst, particularly in the context of the suicide attempt that had just occurred. The analyst decided to provide food immediately, and thinking of the sugar content, told Theresa that she must drink a can of pineapple juice available in the building lunch room. Theresa hesitated, explaining that taking in any food frightened her, as it might give her a sense of being out of control, of being taken over. The analyst reassured her that she did not believe anything bad would happen from drinking the juice, but that if it did, they could talk about it on the spot. There was something about this offer that profoundly affected Theresa. She felt understood, cared for, and, for the first time, protected and somehow not alone in her private struggle at self-regulation.

This incident led to a more direct exploration of Theresa's fear of being taken over by a foreign entity in connection to her fear of both food and medicine intake. It was soon discovered that there was a relationship between her experience of pregnancy with her son, a baby in her uterus, and the feeling of being taken over, an experience she described as disruption, bodily intrusion, and bodily transformation. Over time patient and analyst came to understand that the pregnancy had focused the area of threatened takeover in her pelvic area, that is, her lower abdomen, bladder, urethra, vagina, and anus. During the pregnancy there were times of actual bladder and bowel incontinence accompanied by unknown, unbearable, frightening feelings, which could only be regulated somewhat by intense physical activity and noneating; filling her stomach with food would cause her to become preoccupied with that area, whereas by not eating, keeping her stomach empty, she was able to avoid setting the excruciating process in motion. However, the problem had been compounded more recently, following the birth of her child, because then, with the lowered weight following delivery of the child together with continued avoidance of food, there were periods of great hunger, which in turn led to periodic bingeing, stimulating in the same way the dreaded process. Only slowly did they begin to comprehend that Theresa had lived her entire life without a full range of bodily feelings, and that pregnancy had introduced a heretofore unrealized set of corporeal sensations which had terrified her.

Patient and analyst were thus led back into Theresa's childhood, which until the insight of being numb to feelings in her body, had been only hazy, sugarcoated, and in part quite absent from her memory. Whereas her mother had been described by Theresa when she first came into treatment as perfect, quite different memories of her mother and of her experience in her family began to emerge, but only gradually.

What slowed the process of recovery of memory was an intermittent mutism in her sessions, leading back, then, to recall of a mute adolescence. For long periods, it turned out, Theresa could not talk. She would never talk in school, so that teachers, knowing through her test grades that she had an outstanding grasp of the material, learned never to call on her. At home her parents did not really notice; they saw her instead as a serious student who by her academic interest and achievement made them proud. They thus saw her as involved in her schoolwork, and paid no attention to her lack of communication with them or to her lack of friends. In fact, whatever friendships Theresa was able to develop had been strongly discouraged by her mother.

In the analytic situation, at those times when Theresa would experience the analyst as dangerous, the mute adolescent girl would emerge. Not only could she not talk, but she also felt she could not move her arms easily from a fixed, flexed position. She would hear at those times her own thoughts saying to her, "Don't talk," and she was aware of feeling, "Don't move." These periods in the analysis might dominate the sessions for days at a time, but all Theresa could report of her experience was that she would just find herself in these states for unknown reasons.

In trying to put this picture together, the analyst drew on a statement that Theresa had made earlier quite spontaneously, that her mother would frighten her when she was very young by playing dead at those times when Theresa made some demand on her. Her mother would lie on the floor and remain completely unresponsive to her child's anxious pleas for what seemed like an eternity, until Theresa could learn to sit still, as still as her mother, and try to ignore her own mounting panic. The analyst interpreted to her that in her mute, motionless state on the couch, she might be identifying with her immobile mother, attempting to maintain a kind of primitive contact with her. But although *the analyst* felt better when she could make some sense of Theresa's mute behavior in sessions, it did not seem to help the patient to understand or master that muteness. What did seem to help, however, was an emerging view of her mother as a traumatogenic force in Theresa's life.

Once this newly forming model of Theresa's mother began to take clearer, stronger shape, other memories took on meaning. For example, Theresa remembered her mother's long naps at midday, so that Theresa would often find herself locked out of the house for hours after school, unable to rouse her mother by pounding at the door. She remembered as well her mother's unpredictable mood swings and outbursts of rage with no apparent cause. Or there were her memories of her mother's interminable preparations of simple meals. Canned spaghetti would take literally hours to make. Theresa could put this new set of memories together with her disavowed childhood discovery of stashes of alcohol in the pantry and refrigerator, a current recognition that served to reverberate with images always there but not contextualized until this time in the analysis. With all of these memories available, Theresa could then recall clearly earlier experiences of physical beatings at the hands of her mother. Thus, a completely unanticipated picture of a physically abusive, alcoholic mother emerged, replacing the perfect image that was described by Theresa when treatment began. In turn, this view of Theresa's mother allowed for a deeper exploration of the meanings of the heretofore puzzling lack of physical sensation during childhood, and the new and confusing physical sensations that had been apparent only since the pregnancy began, but that were not understood for some time.

We want to interrupt this case description to point out that in the developmental systems self psychology perspective we are addressing here, a linearly conceived diagnostic category can be recognized to emerge in the clinical setting. In this case, the sense began to grow between patient and analyst that Theresa's was a case of childhood trauma with the depressive phenomena being only an aspect of that linearly conceived etiology and that, in fact, the concomitants of depression in Theresa were better understood as attempts at self-righting through restitutive self-regulation, and as efforts to ward off procedural reexperiencing of traumatic events.

By this point in the analysis, then, the analyst knew that she was dealing with dissociative flashback phenomena in her patient, and she began to think of the DSM-IV category of posttraumatic stress disorder (PTSD). To review briefly some of the highlights of this diagnosis that pertain to Theresa's case, the diagnosis of PTSD includes (1) an exposure to a traumatic event or events that represented a threat to the physical integrity of the self, with a response of intense fear, helplessness, or horror; (2) persistent reexperiencing of the event as recurrent and intrusive distress with dissociative flashback episodes; (3) persistent avoidance of stimuli associated with the trauma, and numbing of general responsiveness; and (4) persistent symptoms of increased arousal, including difficulty in falling or staying asleep, irritability, or outbursts of anger, and difficulty concentrating.

In the case of Theresa, then, the diagnosis of PTSD began to seem the most reasonable hypothesis. Her experiences of muteness in the hours became heightened and more definitive. She felt during those times a generalized excitability, with a total, agitated bodily arousal, including heart racing, fear of dying, inability to move or talk, and of most particular note because it seemed so puzzling, a recurrent, vaginal wetness without vaginal sensation, which occurred during the sessions but was only discovered by Theresa after the session ended.

Investigating this experience of vaginal wetness, combined with the sense of being paralyzed on the couch led to Theresa's reassessment of a particular set of memories of a chronically recurring event that took place during Theresa's adolescence. At bedtime, with her mother apparently in an alcoholic state, and with both mother and Theresa in their nightgowns, Theresa's mother would require her to sit on her lap while her mother caressed her body. Theresa remembered feeling trapped, unable to move, her arms held by her mother rigidly at her sides. When she tried to get up from her mother's lap, her mother would become enraged and would accuse her of being cold and untouchable. Theresa remembered as well that upon being allowed to escape her mother's embrace, the same inexplicable vaginal wetness without vaginal sensation would be apparent to her.

What patient and analyst were confronted with next was a pattern of sudden, unpredictable, rageful outbursts at being forced, as Theresa described it, to lie on the analyst's couch. And indeed, as it turned out, the analyst's unconscious, unformulated countertransference wish to make this patient a more "real" analytic case, and herself, thereby, a more real analyst with her, had contributed significantly to Theresa's sense of being held down and immobilized. The analyst only understood this when it became clear that the couch served Theresa as a retrieval cue for these traumatic events with her mother, currently being revived in the transference where the analyst was now being experienced as the crazy, intrusive, and abandoning mother and Theresa the helpless, abused child. The analyst's part in this enactment was, by subtly insisting on the couch, to repeat the patient's experience of being held down and forced to comply for someone else's purposes, not her own. The immediate experience in the transference of enforced physical intrusion and simultaneous emotional abandonment, not being able to see the analyst's face, provoked in Theresa a powerful annihilation and fragmentation anxiety, a fear of nonexistence. It became clear that the original fear of takeover was a fear of the retraumatizing, intrusive flashback experience.

It came to the analyst spontaneously, then, that Theresa was in the throes of reliving a traumatic experience with her as mother, and that Theresa had at that time no capacity for self-reflection. What she needed in order to stem her rising panic, and to alleviate the fragmentation experience, was to be brought into the present, and what the analyst needed was the sense of direct contact with her, to bring her back into connection with her. Once the analyst understood the gravity of the patient's situation, she could conceive of better ways to be with her when Theresa's dissociative flashback episodes were occurring. To begin with, the analyst discarded any notion of using the couch as a facilitating medium with this patient. Also, she saw the necessity of directly addressing Theresa's position in the here and now by reminding her that the analyst was not her mother and that Theresa was not actually in the past, but rather that the analyst was the analyst in the present, with Theresa, too, in the present. In this context the analyst would express her concern and caring, her dedication, and her conviction that they could get through this together, based on the analyst's own knowledge, in contrast to Theresa's current forgetting, that they had been together for a long time. The analyst told her as well that what Theresa was experiencing was a flashback, a way of remembering very painful experiences, without knowing that she was remembering them.

And so it went whenever these mute panic states would reoccur, with increasing memories recovered that contributed to the development of a fuller picture of sexual and physical abuse from infancy on, abuse that was, incidentally, corroborated later, though only reluctantly, by her mother and other family members. So it went, that is, until one day when the analyst was suddenly confronted with an interruption in her sanguine sense that they were moving forward together. She came to perceive in retrospect that over the past several months she had been losing contact with Theresa, that she was becoming increasingly distant and unreachable, and that none of the analyst's newfound capacities for working with her were successful in keeping the connection in the face of this increasing remoteness on the part of the patient. Remembering that once in the past, during a difficult moment in treatment, Theresa had asked the analyst to hold her hand, the analyst asked Theresa whether she felt it would help if she now held her hand again. Theresa slowly, almost imperceptibly, seemed to agree, although she remained mute and expressionless, so the analyst moved her chair closer and reached out for her hand. This began what evolved into a positive new experience in the analysis, leading to the discovery that when Theresa had seemed so distant, she was actually in a different self state, one that involved being silently removed from this earth. What had made it possible to access this state in communicative, verbal form was the physical contact which had served to keep Theresa aware that she was still on this earth at the same time that she experienced herself as not. She was then able to expose a whole new world of private experience, one that became familiar, and which analyst and patient came to call her "celestial self." In this self state, Theresa's body was experienced quite literally as being used by God for His own very special purposes, which in turn made Theresa herself feel very special, very safe, and very much protected and cared for. They came to understand that as a child Theresa had been able to dissociate in order to protect herself from unbearable, prolonged genital pain inflicted upon her by her mother. It was this capacity for dissociation, used precociously by Theresa, that brought to her self-saving feelings of protection. Only later in her development, when she had acquired symbolic capacities, was this self state symbolically elaborated by her with the narrative that she and the analyst named the celestial self. Although the analyst might have been led to consider a DSM-IV diagnosis of dissociative identity disorder, Theresa was always so present through it all, always herself even when in such a radically altered self state as the celestial experience with God, that it seemed more useful to conceive of her as suffering from multiple self states, remaining somehow always unified as Theresa, and that, indeed, her capacity to dissociate in this way was her salvation. Once this celestial self was discovered, lived with, and lived through in the transference, the connection to the analyst in the present was solidified. A positive new experience with an intimate other evolved between them, as the phenomenon of the dissociative flashback slowly waned and finally disappeared. To provide perspective, Theresa has now been in analysis for 8 years, with

additional work to do, but it is clear that her difficulties are approaching resolution.

We would like at this point to compare briefly these two women
who upon entrance into treatment were both perceived as suffering
from major depression, but who in the treatment situation per se
revealed significant differences in areas that we will now articulate.
We will compare them, first, in terms of the state of the self; second,
in terms of the lived experience postulated for each, including the
ways in which those experiences were predominantly encoded in
memory; third, in terms of the protections for the self evolved by each,
that is, their defensive, self-protective strategies; and fourth, in terms
of the predominant emotions that underlay and organized their depressive presentations.

Emily revealed from the beginning of treatment an integrated self,
with cohesion, agency, affectivity, and historicity in place, whereas
Theresa revealed over time an unintegrated self, disrupted by dissociative self-protective strategies. Self-consolidation for each of these
patients is in process, for Emily, through more hope, and for Theresa,
through a diminishment of dissociative fragmentation. The significance of the analyst for each patient is conceptualized by us as
embodied in the role that analyst serves as both being and providing
a positive new experience for the patient. Through that experience, a
consolidated self is eventually attained, along with a consolidated tie
to the other. This potential for increased consolidation coming
through a positive new experience is exemplified in Emily's case by
the analyst's self-revelation, and in Theresa's case by the analyst's
holding her hand.

The second point we wish to consider in relation to Emily and
Theresa is the nature of the lived experience postulated for each, and
how that lived experience was encoded in memory. Emily's unconscious behavior with the house painter and the antique furniture dealer
was conceptualized by us as procedurally encoded, involving familiar
emotional patterns of withdrawal in the context of self-perceived
interpersonal need. In the analytic session, aspects of her procedural
patterns were observed by her analyst, and then observed to change
as they were converted into declarative form, that is, made conscious
and verbal in the context of a positive new experience. The long
periods of silence, which were at first experienced only as withdrawal
reflecting Emily's hopelessness in regard to getting anything she
needed, became converted into a somewhat more hopeful expectation

that she would be listened to and given to. We anticipate that repeated experiences of having her positive expectations responded to at a procedural level as well as being understood and put into words at a declarative level will enable Emily to change. New, more adaptive behaviors will be encoded by her, and new, more hopeful meanings will be attributed by her to her lived experience.

In Theresa's case, the clinical experience with procedural memory was even more impressive, observed in the dissociative flashback episodes where patterns of fear as well as bodily sensations of pain, intrusion, and takeover were prominent. New responses were extended to Theresa by her analyst, which included the analyst's reassuring presence, feeding, and handholding. These responses provided for the patient alternative ways of experiencing procedurally mediated, self- and mutual-regulatory patterns of being with an other. Also, contextualizing Theresa's experience, and putting words and meanings to that experience, provided for Theresa declaratively mediated, new, positive, and transformative self- and mutual-regulatory patterns of connection. This combination of procedural and declarative exploration, together with positive new experience with an intimate other, permitted Theresa to make sense of, reflect upon, and transform her heretofore mysterious dissociated and fragmented self states so that self-consolidation and consolidation of the intimate attachment to the other could be advanced.

A third component we will address is the self-protective strategies evolved by each. In Emily's case, defensive, self-protective strategies were organized symbolically to protect against a sense of her parents as forever absent and abandoning. She developed a fantasy that she was empty, worthless, and undeserving, experienced through interminable self-criticism, with an unformulated hope that if she were only a better, fuller person, her mother would love and take care of her. This fantasy was split off through disavowal of her conscious knowledge that her mother, and father, too, were in actuality traumatogenic others, emotionally absent, unreachable, and unavailable, that it was her parents who were empty. Despite all this, Emily exhibited even at the beginning of treatment an integrated self, with agency, coherence, affectivity, and historicity more or less in place. The nature of her lived experience and the defensive strategies required for self-protection permitted a relatively more coherent self-structure to be formed. This is in contrast to Theresa, whose self proved to be seriously deficient in agency, coherence, affectivity, and historicity. She was not always the center of her own intentionality; her body was not always experienced as belonging to her; her feelings were often flattened and unavailable, erupting at times in dissociative flashback episodes; and her memory of herself in the past, present, and future was disrupted and fragmented. The nature of Theresa's lived experience was at the hands of a self-shattering other and the defenses required for self-protection under such traumatic circumstances relied primarily on dissociative reactions to maintain whatever integrity of the self was possible. That there was such lived experience in Theresa's case seems evidenced by the self-protective strategies observed clinically. As we have indicated previously, it is now postulated (e.g., Moore, 1994) that dissociation is most often linked with a history of verified physical abuse; further, it is postulated there must be some capacity evolutionarily built into the human being that facilitates dissociation as a defense or self-protection where overwhelming fear arises in the context of life-threatening situations.

We turn now to our fourth point, the predominant emotions that underlay and organized the two patients' depressive presentations. In Emily's case of traumatogenic parental neglect, the predominant core affects underlying her depression were, first, *emptiness*, in which lived experience was laid down in the form of self-regulatory, mutual-regulatory, and interpersonal interactions of self with other wherein that other was absent or depressed, and the interactions were encoded both procedurally and symbolically; and, second, *aloneness*, which was at first only procedurally encoded, and subsequently elaborated with fantasies and meanings at the point in development when such elaborations in fantasy became possible, so that Emily created the idea that she was so empty and unworthy that no parent or any other could ever love her or respond to her. With Theresa, a case of childhood trauma, the predominant core affects underlying her depression were profound *annihilation* and *fragmentation anxiety* in which lived experience was laid down in the form of self-regulatory, mutual-regulatory, and interpersonal interactions of self with other wherein that other was self-shattering and intensely traumatogenic, and the interactions were encoded on both procedural and symbolic levels.

In both cases suicidal ideation was prominent. With Emily, the self-destructive feelings were maintained at the ideational level, designed to escape feelings of unbearable emptiness and aloneness. With Theresa, there was an actual suicide attempt, designed to escape the unbearable reliving of the trauma, to end the pain once and for all. Both experienced unbearable pain, but because Emily's self was coherent and cohesive, she could maintain a connection with a healthier aspect of herself, the need to protect her child. But with Theresa, the self was shattered, leaving her, in the face of the dissociative flashback episodes, with no way of reclaiming those split-off, healthier aspects of her self, and no way to picture a future in which her suffering might be relieved. The continuity of the self as containing a future was unavailable to Theresa, whereas for Emily a future could be imagined, at least for that part of herself that would remain alive in her child.

We end with a conclusion about depression as it presents in the clinical setting. We see depression as a complex state best understood as arising from and embedded within a system influenced by many factors. These factors include the state of the self, whether integrated or unintegrated, consolidated or unconsolidated; the nature of the lived experience, whether the trauma is of neglect, abuse, or some combination; the ways in which lived experience is encoded, especially whether symbolized or not; the nature of the self-protective strategies evolved by the self; and, finally, the predominant emotions underlying and organizing the depressive presentation.

With this consideration of depression in two adult patients, we end our discussion of the clinical situation across the lifespan. We will turn now to a final look at the application of our central concepts. With Emily, the analysis began in a fixed old self with old other patient–analyst relational configuration, with some progress toward an old self with new other configuration emergent as the analyst was able to serve effectively in a self-transforming dimension of intimacy. In the session we present, the analyst initiates an interpersonal-sharing experience, with some success, patient and analyst enjoying together a moment of shared humanity and a beginning regulation of the patient's affect of profound shame. However, Emily remains mainly in the self-transforming dimension of intimacy in an old–old configuration, with self-integration intact but with self-consolidation lacking. Positive new experience is achieved in the dyad only slowly, the grip of the past being strong and tenacious. An ongoing security and intimate attachment still eludes this patient, with an avoidant attachment pattern still predominant.

As for Theresa, the analysis began in an old self with new other relational pattern, dropping back into an old self with old other relational pattern when severely traumatic flashback states emerged. Both self-integration and self-consolidation were compromised in such periods. Once the analyst was successful in finding ways to connect with her, particularly through using an interpersonal-sharing dimension of intimacy that also had self-transforming effects, the patient could move for some periods to a new self with new other patient–analyst relational configuration. The disorganized attachment pattern was replaced at such times by a secure attachment and a concomitant consolidation of the self. Intimate attachment and positive new experience were achieved and in fact notable in the dyad. The trajectory of developmental progression appears to be clearly in the direction of a more stable new self with a new other relational configuration.

References

Ainsworth, M. (1982). Attachment, retrospect and prospect. In C. Parkes & J. Stevenson-Hinde (Eds.), *The place of attachments in human behavior* (pp. 3–31). New York: Basic Books.

Ainsworth, M. (1985). I. Patterns of infant–mother attachment: Antecedents and effects on development, and II. Attachments across the lifespan. *Bulletin of the New York Academy of Medicine, 61*, 771–791; 791–812.

American Psychiatric Association. (1994). *Diagnostic and statistical manual of mental disorders* (4th ed.). Washington, DC: Author.

Bacal, H. (1985). Optimal responsiveness and the therapeutic process. In A. Goldberg (Ed.), *Progress in self psychology* (Vol. 1, pp. 202–227). New York: Guilford Press.

Bair, D. (1990). *Simone de Beauvoir: A biography.* New York: Summit Books.

Beebe, B., & Lachmann, F. M. (1992). The contribution of mother–infant mutual influence to the origin of self and object representations. In N. Skolnick & S. Warshaw (Eds.), *Relational perspectives in psychoanalysis* (pp. 83–117). Hillsdale, NJ: Analytic Press.

Benedek, T. (1959). Parenthood as a developmental phase. In *Psychoanalytic investigation: Selected papers* (pp. 378–394). New York: Quadrangle Press, 1979.

Bloch, H. (1995). *Adolescent development: Psychopathology and treatment.* Madison, CT: International Universities Press.

Bowlby, J. (1969). *Attachment.* New York: Basic Books.

Bowlby, J. (1973). *Separation.* New York: Basic Books.

Bowlby, J. (1988). *A secure base.* New York: Basic Books.

Bowlby, J. (1989). *Loss.* New York: Basic Books.

Bowlby, J. (1990). *Attachment theory.* Lecture presented at the Continuing Education Series of UCLA, London.

Brandchaft, B. (1994). *Structures of pathological accommodation.* Unpublished manuscript.

Brenner, C. (1982). *The mind in conflict.* New York: International Universities Press.

Bruner, S. (1990). *Acts of meaning.* Cambridge, MA: Harvard University Press.

Carroll, L. (1865). *Alice's adventures in Wonderland.* New York: Macmillan.

Cath, S. H. (1985). Clinical vignettes: A range of grandparental experiences. *Journal of the Geriatric Society, 23*, 57–68.

Cavell, M. (1993). *The psychoanalytic mind: From Freud to philosophy.* Cambridge, MA: Harvard University Press.

Clyman, R. (1991). The procedural organization of emotions: A contribution from cognitive science to the psychoanalytic theory of therapeutic action. *Journal of the American Psychological Association, 39*, 349–382.

Cocks, G. (1994). *Curve of life: Correspondence of Heinz Kohut.* Chicago: University of Chicago Press.

Cramer, B. G. (1992). *The importance of being baby.* Reading, MA: Addison-Wesley.

Damasio, A. (1994). *Descartes' error: Emotions, reason and the human brain.* New York: G. P. Putnam's Sons.

Davidson, D. (1986). A coherence theory of truth and knowledge. In E. LePore (Ed.), *Truth and interpretation: Perspectives on the philosophy of Donald Davidson.* Oxford: Blackwell.

Davies, J. M., & Frawley, M. G. (1994). *Treating the adult survivor of childhood abuse: A psychoanalytic perspective.* New York: Basic Books.

Doolittle, H. (1984). *Tribute to Freud: Writing on the wall* (2nd ed.). New York: Direction–Norton.

Edelman, G. (1992). *Bright air, brilliant fire: On the matter of the mind.* New York: Basic Books.

Eliot, G. (1874/1876). *Daniel Deronda.* New York: New American Library, 1979.

Erickson, M. (1993). Rethinking Oedipus: An evolutionary perspective of incest avoidance. *American Journal of Psychiatry, 150*, 411–416.

Erikson, E. H. (1950). *Childhood and society.* New York: W. W. Norton.

Ferber, R. (1985). *Solve your child's sleep problems.* New York: Simon & Schuster.

Fonagy, P., Steele, H., & Steele, M. (1991). Maternal representations of attachment during pregnancy predict the organization of infant–mother attachment at one year of age. *Child Development, 62*, 891–905.

Fonagy, P., Steele, M., Steele, H., Moran, G. S., & Higgitt, A. C. (1991). The capacity for understanding mental states: The reflective self in parent and child and its significance for security of attachment. *Infant Mental Health Journal, 12*(3), 201–218.

Fosshage, J. (in press). Listening/experiencing perspectives and the quest for a facilitating responsiveness. *Progress in Self Psychology, 13.*

Freud, A. (1966). *Normality and pathology in childhood: Assessments of development.* New York: International Universities Press.

Freud, S. (1899). Screen memories. *Standard Edition, 3*, 301–322.

Freud, S. (1905). Three essays on the theory of sexuality. *Standard Edition, 7*, 125–244.

Freud, S. (1912). The dynamics of transference. *Standard Edition, 12*, 99–120.

Friedman, R. (1988). *Male homosexuality: A contemporary psychoanalytic perspective.* New Haven, CT: Yale University Press.

Furman, R. (1996). Methylphenidate and "ADHD" in Europe and the USA. *Child Analysis, 7,* 132–145.

Galatzer-Levy, R. M., & Cohler, B. J. (1993). *The essential other: A developmental psychology of the self.* New York: Basic Books.

Gales, M. E. (1978). *Mother–infant bonding.* Grand Rounds presentation, University of California, Los Angeles.

Gill, M. (1982). *Analysis of transference* (Vol. 1). Madison, CT: International Universities Press.

Goldberg, A. (1978). *The psychology of the self: A casebook.* New York: International Universities Press.

Goldberg, A. (1990). *The prisonhouse of psychoanalysis.* Hillsdale, NJ: Analytic Press.

Goodman, S. (Ed). (1977). *Psychoanalytic education and research: The current solution and future possibilities.* New York: International Universities Press.

Greenson, R. R. (1967). *The technique and practice of psychoanalysis* (Vol. 1). New York: International Universities Press.

Grigsby, J., & Hartlaub, G. H. (1994). Procedural learning and the development and stability of character. *Perceptual and Motor Skills, 79,* 355–370.

Hamburg, D. (1977). Toward a strategy for healthy adolescent development. *American Journal of Psychiatry, 154,* 6–12.

Harlow, H. F., & Harlow, M. K. (1965). The affectual systems. In A. M. Shrier, H. F. Harlow, & F. Stollnitz (Eds.), *Behavior of nonhuman primates* (Vol. 2). New York: Academic Press.

Hartmann, H. (1950). Comments on the psychoanalytic theory of the ego. In *Essays on ego psychology* (pp. 4–5). New York: International Universities Press, 1964.

Hawking, S. W. (1988). *A brief history of time: From the big bang to black holes.* New York: Bantam Books.

Henry, O. (W. S. Porter). (1984). The gift of the Magi. In *41 stories by O. Henry* (pp. 65–70). New York: Signet Classics. (Original work published 1906).

Herman, J. L. (1992). *Trauma and recovery: The aftermath of violence—From domestic abuse to political terror.* New York: Basic Books.

Karen, R. (1990, February). Becoming attached: What experiences in infancy will enable children to thrive emotionally and to come to feel that the world of people is a positive place? *Atlantic Monthly,* p. 49.

Kernberg, O. (1988). Object relations theory in classical practice. *Psychoanalytic Quarterly, 57,* 481–504.

Kohut, H. (1968). Forms and transformations of narcissism. *Journal of the American Psychoanalytic Association, 14*(2), 243–272.

Kohut, H. (1977). *The restoration of the self.* New York: International Universities Press.

Kohut, H. (1984). *How does analysis cure?* (A. Goldberg & P. Stepansky, Eds.). Chicago: University of Chicago Press.

Kris, E. (1956). The recovery of childhood memories in psychoanalysis. *Psychoanalytic Study of the Child, 11,* 54–88.

Lichtenberg, J. (1989). *Psychoanalysis and motivation.* Hillsdale, NJ: Analytic Press.

Lichtenberg, J., Lachmann, F., & Fosshage, J. (1992). *Self and motivational systems: Toward a theory of psychoanalytic technique.* Hillsdale, NJ: Analytic Press.

Lipton, S. D. (1977). The advantages of Freud's technique as shown in his analysis of the Rat Man. *International Journal of Psycho-Analysis, 58,* 255–273.

Loewald, H. W. (1960). On the therapeutic action of psycho-analyses. *International Journal of Psycho-Analysis, 15,* 127–159.

Lorenz, K. Z. (1935). Der Kumpan in der Umvelt des Vogels. In C. H. Schiller (Ed.), *Instinctual behavior.* New York: International Universities Press, 1957.

Lyons-Ruth, K. (1992). Rapprochement or approchement: Mahler's theory reconsidered from the vantage point of recent research on early attachment relationships. *Psychoanalytic Psychology, 8,* 1–23.

Mahler, M. S., Pine, F., & Bergman, A. (1975). *The psychological birth of the human infant.* New York: Basic Books.

Main, M., & Goldwyn, R. (1985). *Adult attachment classification and rating system.* Unpublished manuscript, University of California at Berkeley.

Main, M., & Hesse, E. (1992). Disorganized/disoriented infant behavior in the Strange Situation, lapses in the monitoring of reasoning and discourse during the parent's adult attachment interview, and dissociative states. In M. Ammaniti & D. Stern (Eds.), *Attachment and psychoanalysis.* Rome: Guis, Laterz & Figli.

Main, M., & Solomon, J. (1986). Discovery of an insecure disorganized/disoriented attachment patter. In T. B. Brazelton & M. W. Yogman (Eds.), *Affective development in infancy.* Norwood, NJ: Ablex.

Main, M., & Solomon, J. (1990). Procedures for identifying infants as disorganized-disoriented during the Ainsworth Strange Situation. In M. Greenberg, D. Cicchetti, & E. M. Cummings (Eds.), *Attachment in preschool years: Theory, research and intervention* (pp. 121–160). Chicago: University of Chicago Press.

McDonough, S. C. (1993). Interaction guidance: Understanding and treating early infant–caregiver relationship disorders. In C. M. Zeanah (Ed.), *Handbook of infant mental health* (pp. 414–426). New York: Guilford Press.

Meissner, W. (1991). *What is effective in psychoanalytic therapy: The move from interpretation to relation.* Northvale, NJ: Jason Aronson.

Modell, A. H. (1988). The centrality of the psychoanalytic setting and the changing aims of treatment: A perspective from a theory of object relations. *Psychoanalytic Quarterly, 57,* 577–596.

Moore, M. S. (1994, January). *A presentation on traumatic attachments.* Meeting of the Institute of Contemporary Psychoanalysis, Los Angeles.

Offer, D. (1969). *The psychological world of the teenager: A study of normal adolescent boys.* New York: Basic Books.

Ornstein, P., & Ornstein, A. (1980). Formulating interpretations in child psychoanalysis. *International Journal of Psycho-Analysis, 61,* 203–211.

Piaget, J. (1954). *The construction of reality in the child.* New York: Basic Books.

Piaget, J. (1962). *Play, dreams, and imitation in childhood.* New York: Norton.

Piaget, J., & Inhelder, B. (1969). *The psychology of the child.* New York: Basic Books.

Person, E. (1991, June). Paper presented at the panel "On Intimacy and Romantic Love" at the Los Angeles Child Development Center, Los Angeles.

Pine, F. (1990). *Drive, ego, and self: A synthesis for clinical work.* New York: Basic Books.

Pynoos, R. S., & Eth, S. (1985). Developmental perspective in psychic trauma in childhood. In C. R. Figley (Ed.), *Trauma and its wake.* New York: Brunner/Mazel.

Rapoport, D. (1960a). Psychoanalysis as a developmental psychology. In M. M. Gill (Ed.), *The collected papers of David Rapaport* (pp. 820–853). New York: Basic Books.

Rapaport, D. (1960b). On the psychoanalytic theory of motivation. In M. M. Gill (Ed.), *The collected papers of David Rapaport* (pp. 853–915). New York: Basic Books.

Robertson, J., & Robertson, J. (Directors), & Tavistock Institute of Human Relations (Producer). (1969). *Young children in brief separation: Film No. 3. John 17 months for 9 days in a residential nursery* [Film]. (Available from New York University Film Library).

Robertson, J., & Bowlby, J. (1952). Responses of young children to separation from their mothers. *Courier Centre Internationale Enfance, 2,* 131–142.

Sander, L. W. (1962). Issues in early mother–child interaction. *Journal of the American Academy of Child Psychiatry, 1,* 141–166.

Sander, L. W. (1964). Adaptive relationships in early mother–child interaction. *Journal of the American Academy of Child Psychiatry, 3,* 231–234.

Schlessinger, N., & Robbins, F. (1983). *A developmental view of the psychoanalytic process.* New York: International Universities Press.

Seleznick, S. (1965). Paper presented at the panel on countertransference at the joint meeting of the Los Angeles Psychoanalytic Institute and the Southern California Psychoanalytic Institute, Los Angeles.

Settlage, C. F., Curtix, Z., Lozoff, M., Siberschatz, G., & Simberg, E. (1988). Conceptualizing adult development. *Journal of the American Psychoanalytic Association, 36,* 347–370.

Shane, E., Gales, M., & Shane, M. (1995). *A developmental systems approach to depression.* Paper presented at a symposium on women and depression, Georgetown University, Washington, DC.

Shane, E., & Shane, M. (1984). *Review of the complete published works of Margaret Mahler*. Paper presented at the Mahler Study Group, New York.

Shane, E., & Shane, M. (1997). Intimacy, boundaries and countertransference in the analytic relationship. *Psychoanalytic Inquiry, 7,* 69–89.

Shane, M. (1968). *The adult toy*. Paper presented at the Western Regional Psychoanalytic Meeting, San Diego, June, and the American Psychoanalytic Meeting, New York, December.

Shane, M. (1977). A rationale for teaching analytic technique based on a developmental orientation and approach. *International Journal of Psycho-Analysis, 58,* 95–103.

Shane, M. (1980). Essays on the developmental orientation in psychoanalysis: Countertransference and the developmental orientation and approach. *Psychoanalysis and Comtemporary Thought,3(2).*

Shane, M. (1991). Selfobject or self-regulating other. *Progress in Self Psychology, 7,* 31–35.

Shane, M., & Shane, E. (1989). The struggle for otherhood: Implications for development in adulthood. *Psychoanalytic Inquiry, 9,* 466–481.

Shane, M., & Shane, E. (1993). Self psychology after Kohut: One theory or many? *Journal of the American Psychological Association, 43,* 372–377.

Shane, M., & Shane, E. (1996). Self psychology in search of the optimal: A consideration of optimal responsiveness, optimal provision, optimal gratification and optimal restraint in clinical situation. *Progress in Self Psychology, 12,* 37–54.

Slap, J. W., & Slap-Shelton, L. (1991). *The schema in clinical psychoanalysis*. Hillsdale, NJ: Analytic Press.

Socarides, D. D., & Stolorow, R. (1984–1985). Affects and selfobjects. *Annual of Psychoanalysis, 12/13,* 105–119.

Spitz, R. (1946). Anaclitic depression. *Psychoanalytic Study of the Child, 2,*313–342.

Spitz, R., & Cobliner, W. (1965). *The first year of life*. New York: International Universities Press.

Sroufe, L. A. (1996). *Emotional development: The organization of emotional life in the early years*. New York: Cambridge University Press.

Stein, M. (1981). The unobjectionable part of the transference. *Journal of the American Psychoanalytic Association, 29,* 869–892.

Stern, D. N. (1985). *The interpersonal world of the infant*. New York: Basic Books.

Stern, D. N. (1995). *The motherhood constellation: A unified view of parent–infant psychotherapies*. New York: Basic Books.

Stoller, R. J. (1975). *Perversion*. New York: Pantheon.

Stolorow, R. (1997). Dynamic, dyadic intersubjective systems: An evolving paradigm for psychoanalysis. *Psychoanalytic Psychology, 14,* 337–346.

Stolorow, R., & Atwood, G. (1992). *Context of being: The intersubjective foundations of psychological life*. Hillsdale, NJ: Analytic Press.

Stolorow, R., Brandchaft, B., & Atwood, G. (1987). *Psychoanalytic treatment: An intersubjective approach.* Hillsdale, NJ: Analytic Press.

Strachey, J. (1934). The nature of the therapeutic action of psychoanalysis. *International Journal of Psycho-Analysis, 15,* 127–159.

Strenger, C. (1991). *Between hermeneutics and science.* New York: International Universities Press.

Terman, D. (1988). Optimal frustration: Structuralization and the therapeutic process. *Progress in Self Psychology, 4,* 113–125.

Thelan, E., & Smith, L. B. (1994). *A dynamic systems approach to the development of cognition and action.* Cambridge, MA: MIT Press.

Tolpin, M. (1986). The self and its selfobjects: A different baby. In A. I. Goldberg (Ed.), *Progress in self psychology* (Vol. 2, pp. 113–125). Hillsdale, NJ: Analytic Press.

Tolpin, P. (1985). The primacy of the preservation of self. In A. I. Goldberg (Ed.), *Progress in self psychology* (Vol. 1, pp. 83–87). New York: Guilford Press.

Tyson, P., & Tyson, R. (1990). *Psychoanalytic theories of development: An integration.* New Haven, CT: Yale University Press.

Uzgiris, I. C. (1973). Patterns of vocal and gestural imitation in infants. In L. J. Stone, H. T. Smith, & L. B. Murphy (Eds.), *The competent infant* (pp. 599–604). New York: Basic Books.

van der Kolk, B. A., McFarlane, A. C., & Weisaeth, L. (Eds.). (1996). *Traumatic stress: The effects of overwhelming experience on mind, body, and society.* New York: Guilford Press.

Winnicott, D. W. (1960). Ego distortion in terms of true and false self. In *The maturational process and the facilitating environment* (pp. 140–152). London: Hogarth.

Winnicott, D. W. (1971). *Playing and reality.* New York: Basic Books.

Wolf, E. S. (1988). *Treating the self: Elements of clinical self psychology.* New York: Guilford Press.

Wright, A. (1996). *Infant psychiatry: Models of intervention for infants and families.* Paper presented at the Menniger conference: At-Risk Infants: Assessment and Treatment in Multi-risk Families, Topeka, Kansas.

Index